Eating Disorders: Part I

Editors

HARRY A. BRANDT
STEVEN F. CRAWFORD

PSYCHIATRIC CLINICS
OF NORTH AMERICA

www.psych.theclinics.com

Consulting Editor
HARSH K. TRIVEDI

March 2019 • Volume 42 • Number 1

ELSEVIER

1600 John F. Kennedy Boulevard • Suite 1800 • Philadelphia, Pennsylvania, 19103-2899

http://www.theclinics.com

PSYCHIATRIC CLINICS OF NORTH AMERICA Volume 42, Number 1
March 2019 ISSN 0193-953X, ISBN-13: 978-0-323-67876-6

Editor: Lauren Boyle
Developmental Editor: Kristen Helm

Psychiatric Clinics of North America (ISSN 0193-953X) is published quarterly by Elsevier Inc., 360 Park Avenue South, New York, NY 10010-1710. Months of issue are March, June, September, and December. Business and Editorial Offices: 1600 John F. Kennedy Blvd., Suite 1800, Philadelphia, PA 19103-2899. Periodicals postage paid at New York, NY and additional mailing offices. Subscription prices are $332.00 per year (US individuals), $699.00 per year (US institutions), $100.00 per year (US students/residents), $406.00 per year (Canadian individuals), $462.00 per year (international individuals), $880.00 per year (Canadian & international institutions), and $220.00 per year (Canadian & international students/residents). Foreign air speed delivery is included in all *Clinics'* subscription prices. All prices are subject to change without notice. **POSTMASTER:** Send address changes to *Psychiatric Clinics of North America*, Elsevier Health Sciences Division, Subscription Customer Service, 3251 Riverport Lane, Maryland Heights, MO 63043. **Customer Service: 1-800-654-2452 (US). From outside the United States, call 1-314-447-8871. Fax: 1-314-447-8029. E-mail: journalscustomerservice-usa@elsevier.com (for print support)** and **journalsonline support-usa@elsevier.com (for online support).**

Reprints. For copies of 100 or more, of articles in this publication, please contact the Commercial Reprints Department, Elsevier Inc., 360 Park Avenue South, New York, New York 10010-1710. Tel.: 212-633-3874, Fax: 212-633-3820, E-mail: reprints@elsevier.com.

Psychiatric Clinics of North America is covered in *MEDLINE/PubMed (Index Medicus), Current Contents/Social and Behavioral Sciences, Social Science Citation Index, Embase/Excerpta Medica,* and PsycINFO.

Contributors

CONSULTING EDITOR

HARSH K. TRIVEDI, MD, MBA
President & Chief Executive Officer, Sheppard Pratt Health System, Baltimore, Maryland, USA

EDITORS

HARRY A. BRANDT, MD
Co-Director, Center for Eating Disorders at Sheppard Pratt, Chief, Department of Psychiatry, University of Maryland, St. Joseph Medical Center, Clinical Associate Professor, University of Maryland School of Medicine, Towson, Maryland, USA

STEVEN F. CRAWFORD, MD
Co-Director, Center for Eating Disorders at Sheppard Pratt, Assistant Chief, Department of Psychiatry, University of Maryland, St. Joseph Medical Center, Clinical Associate Professor, University of Maryland School of Medicine, Towson, Maryland, USA

AUTHORS

EVELYN ATTIA, MD
Professor, Department of Psychiatry, New York State Psychiatric Institute, Columbia University Irving Medical Center, New York, New York, USA

JEHANNINE AUSTIN, PhD, CCGC/CGC
Research Chair in Translational Psychiatric Genomics, Associate Professor, Departments of Psychiatry and Medical Genetics, University of British Columbia, Vancouver, British Columbia, Canada

LAURA A. BERNER, PhD
Postdoctoral Scholar, Department of Psychiatry, University of California, San Diego, Eating Disorders Center for Treatment and Research, San Diego, California, USA

LAUREN E. BLAKE, MS, NSF
Graduate Research Fellow, Department of Human Genetics, University of Chicago, Chicago, Illinois, USA

RACHEL BRYANT-WAUGH, BSc, MSc, DPhil
Honorary Consultant Clinical Psychologist, Department of Child and Adolescent Mental Health, Great Ormond Street Hospital for Children NHS Foundation Trust, Honorary Senior Lecturer, Population, Policy and Practice Programme, University College London Institute of Child Health, London, United Kingdom

CYNTHIA M. BULIK, PhD
Distinguished Professor, Department of Psychiatry, UNC Chapel Hill, Professor, Department of Nutrition, University of North Carolina, Chapel Hill, North Carolina, USA; Professor, Department of Medical Epidemiology and Biostatistics, Karolinska Institutet, Stockholm, Sweden

BEATE HERPERTZ-DAHLMANN, MD
Department of Child and Adolescent Psychiatry, Psychotherapy and Psychosomatics, University Hospital, RWTH University Aachen, Aachen, Germany

ANJA HILBERT, PhD
Professor of Behavioral Medicine, Integrated Research and Treatment Center Adiposity Diseases, Department of Medical Psychology and Medical Sociology, Department of Psychosomatic Medicine and Psychotherapy, University of Leipzig Medical Center, Leipzig, Germany

CAROL KAN, MRCPsych, PhD
Section of Eating Disorders, Clinical Lecturer, Department of Psychological Medicine, Institute of Psychiatry, Psychology and Neuroscience, King's College London, London, United Kingdom

DEBRA K. KATZMAN, MD, FRCPC
Division of Adolescent Medicine, Professor, Department of Pediatrics, Director, Health Science Research, Faculty of Medicine, Senior Associate Scientist, Research Institute, The Hospital for Sick Children, University of Toronto, Toronto, Ontario, Canada

SIÂN A. McLEAN, PhD
Research Fellow, Institute for Health and Sport, Victoria University, Melbourne, Victoria, Australia

MARK L. NORRIS, MD, FRCPC
Division of Adolescent Medicine, Associate Professor, Department of Pediatrics, The Children's Hospital of Eastern Ontario (CHEO), University of Ottawa, Clinical Investigator, CHEO Research Institute, Ottawa, Ontario, Canada

SUSAN J. PAXTON, PhD
Emeritus Professor, Department of Psychology and Counselling, School of Psychology and Public Health, La Trobe University, Melbourne, Victoria, Australia

JOCHEN SEITZ, MD
Department of Child and Adolescent Psychiatry, Psychotherapy and Psychosomatics, University Hospital, RWTH University Aachen, Aachen, Germany

JOANNA E. STEINGLASS, MD
Associate Professor of Clinical Psychiatry, Department of Psychiatry, New York State Psychiatric Institute, Columbia University Irving Medical Center, New York, New York, USA

JANET TREASURE, FRCPsych, FRCP, PhD
Professor of Psychiatry, Eating Disorders Unit, South London and Maudsley NHS Foundation Trust, London, United Kingdom

STEFANIE TRINH, MSc
Institute for Neuroanatomy, University Hospital, RWTH University Aachen, Aachen, Germany

KELLY M. VITOUSEK, PhD
Associate Professor, Department of Psychology, University of Hawai'i at Mānoa, Honolulu, Hawaii, USA

TRACEY D. WADE, PhD
Matthew Flinders Distinguished Professor of Psychology, School of Psychology, Flinders University, Adelaide, South Australia, Australia

ALLISON F. WAGNER, MA
Graduate Student, Department of Psychology, University of Hawai'i at Mānoa, Honolulu, Hawaii, USA

B. TIMOTHY WALSH, MD
New York State Psychiatric Institute, Department of Psychiatry, Columbia University Irving Medical Center, New York, USA

RUTH STRIEGEL WEISSMAN, PhD
Professor of Psychology, Walter A. Crowell Professor of the Social Sciences, Emerita, Wesleyan University, Middletown, Connecticut, USA

NANCY ZUCKER, PhD
Associate Professor, Departments of Psychiatry and Behavioral Sciences, and Psychology and Neuroscience, Duke School of Medicine, Duke University, Director, Duke Center for Eating Disorders, Durham, North Carolina, USA

Contents

Eating Disorders Overview of Diagnostic Considerations

> The *Diagnostic and Statistical Manual of Mental Disorders (Fifth Edition)* for 6 feeding and eating disorders were published in 2013 and were notable for officially recognizing binge-eating disorder and for articulating criteria for avoidant/restrictive food intake disorder. The criteria and the rationale for them are briefly described, and current and future challenges are discussed.

> Recent advances in the understanding of aetiologic elements underlying anorexia nervosa have provided valuable insights and are transforming the way this illness is treated. The aim of this article is to consider how neuropsychological understanding and new research can be used to develop a more individualized and personalized approach in the management of this serious illness.

> Estimates of lifetime bulimia nervosa (BN) range from 4% to 6.7% across studies. There has been a decrease in the presentation of BN in primary care but an increase in disordered eating not meeting full diagnostic criteria. Regardless of diagnostic status, disordered eating is associated with long-term significant impairment to both physical and mental quality of life, and BN is associated with a significantly higher likelihood of self-harm, suicide, and death. Assessment should adopt a motivationally enhancing stance given the high level of ambivalence associated with BN. Cognitive behavior therapy specific to eating disorders outperforms other active psychological comparisons.

> Binge-eating disorder (BED), first included as a diagnostic entity in the Diagnostic and Statistical Manual of Mental Disorders Fifth Edition, is characterized by recurrent episodes of binge eating without regular compensatory behaviors to prevent weight gain. With a complex multifactorial etiology, BED is the most frequent eating disorder co-occuring with significant psychopathology, mental and physical comorbidity, obesity, and life

impairment. Despite its significance, BED is not sufficiently diagnosed or treated. Evidence-based treatments for BED include psychotherapy and structured self-help treatment, with cognitive-behavioral therapy as most well-established approach, and pharmacotherapy with lisdexamfetamine as FDA approved medication with a limitation of use.

Avoidant restrictive food intake disorder (ARFID) is a rearticulated eating disorder diagnosis in the *Diagnostic and Statistical Manual of Mental Disorders* (fifth edition) (*DSM-5*), published in 2013. The purpose of this article is to review what is known about ARFID; specifically outline the *DSM-5* diagnostic criteria; review the epidemiology; describe the clinical characteristics of patients with this disorder; and discuss evolving treatment approaches. Although this disorder occurs across the lifespan, the focus of recent research has been primarily in children and adolescents with ARFID. Therefore, most of this article is devoted to children and adolescents with ARFID.

Etiological Considerations

Anorexia nervosa (AN), bulimia nervosa (BN), and binge-eating disorder (BED) are heritable conditions that are influenced by both genetic and environmental factors. Recent genome-wide association (GWA) studies of AN have identified specific genetic loci implicated in AN, and genetic correlations have implicated both psychiatric and metabolic factors in its origin. No GWAS have been performed for BN or BED. Genetic counseling is an important tool and can aid families and patients in understanding risk for these illnesses.

Anorexia nervosa and bulimia nervosa are characterized by severely restricted intake, binge eating, and compensatory behaviors like self-induced vomiting. The neurobiological underpinnings of these maladaptive behaviors are poorly understood, but the application of cognitive neuroscience and neuroimaging to eating disorders has begun to elucidate their pathophysiology. Specifically, this review focuses on 3 areas that suggest paths forward: reward, cognitive and behavioral control, and decision making. Understanding the brain-based mechanisms that promote and maintain these often chronic symptoms could guide the development of new and more effective treatments.

Growing interest exists in the association of gut bacteria with diseases, such as diabetes, obesity, inflammatory bowel disease, and psychiatric disorders. Gut microbiota influence the fermentation of nutrients, body-weight regulation, gut permeability, hormones, inflammation, immunology, and behavior (gut-brain axis). Regarding anorexia nervosa (AN), altered microbial diversity and taxa abundance were found and associated with depressive, anxious, and eating disorder symptoms. Potential mechanisms involve increased gut permeability, low-grade inflammation, autoantibodies, and reduced brain cell neogenesis and learning. Gut microbiome is strongly influenced by refeeding practices. Microbiota-modulating strategies like nutritional interventions or psychobiotics application could become relevant additions to AN treatment.

Personality variables have long been implicated in the onset and maintenance of eating disorders, as well as in symptom divergence between anorexia nervosa and bulimia nervosa. Clinical observations are broadly supported by the data, with restricting anorexia nervosa associated with higher levels of constraint and Persistence, and binge-purge behaviors linked to the tendency to take impulsive action when emotionally distressed. Considerable heterogeneity is found within diagnostic categories, however, suggesting that different personality structures may predispose individuals to develop disordered eating through alternative pathways.

Most theories emphasize the role of sociocultural factors in the etiology of eating disorders (EDs). This article uses a broad search strategy to identify current etiologic studies. Women with an ED outnumber men in each diagnosis, but gender differences vary by diagnosis. Men are underrepresented in study samples, and information about variable risk factors in men is sparse. Findings suggest transdiagnostic risk factors and disorder-specific risk factors. Extracting data from population-based registers represents a major advance. Novel analytic approaches suggest complex pathways to ED. Although used in several studies, reliance on a transdiagnostic ED category (vs diagnosis-specific groupings) is premature.

Other Topics

Body dissatisfaction is a risk factor for development of eating disorders and represents a core psychopathologic feature of eating disorders. Prevention and treatment interventions address established risk and maintaining factors for body dissatisfaction: appearance pressures, internalization of appearance ideals, upward appearance comparison, avoidance and checking, and body disparagement. It is essential to address body dissatisfaction within eating disorders treatment to improve outcomes and reduce risk of relapse. Future directions in research and treatment aim to reach populations increasingly recognized as in need, including children, men, and individuals at higher weights, with the ultimate goal of reducing the significant distress associated with body dissatisfaction.

Rachel Bryant-Waugh

This article provides an update based on recently published literature and expert consensus on the current state of knowledge regarding feeding and eating disorders in children aged 2 to 12 years. It covers the 6 main diagnostic categories—pica, rumination disorder, avoidant/restrictive food intake disorder, anorexia nervosa, bulimia nervosa, and binge eating disorder—discussing issues and findings specific to this age group. It highlights the need for ongoing research in a number of key areas, to include improved understanding of etiologic pathways, characterization of presenting disorders, and the development of standardized evidence-based assessment tools and treatment interventions.

PSYCHIATRIC CLINICS OF NORTH AMERICA

FORTHCOMING ISSUES

June 2019
Eating Disorders: Part II
Harry A. Brandt and
Steven F. Crawford, *Editors*

September 2019
Professional Development for Psychiatrists
Howard Y. Liu and Donald Hilty, *Editors*

December 2019
Integrating Technology into 21st Century Psychiatry: Telemedicine, Social Media, and other Technologies
James H. Shore, *Editor*

RECENT ISSUES

December 2018
Borderline Personality Disorder
Frank Yeomans and Kenneth N. Levy, *Editors*

September 2018
Neuromodulation
Scott T. Aaronson and
Noah S. Philip, *Editors*

June 2018
Psychodynamic Psychiatry
Thomas N. Franklin, *Editor*

SERIES OF RELATED INTEREST

Child and Adolescent Psychiatric Clinics of North America
Neurologic Clinics

THE CLINICS ARE AVAILABLE ONLINE!
Access your subscription at:
www.theclinics.com

PSYCHIATRIC CLINICS OF
NORTH AMERICA
EATING DISORDERS

FORTHCOMING ISSUES

Eating Disorders: Part II
Harry A. Brandt, and
Steven F. Crawford, Editors

September 2019
Professional Development for Psychiatrists
Howard Y. Liu and Donald Hilty, Editors

December 2019
Integrating Technology into 21st Century
Psychiatry: Telemedicine, Social Media,
and other Technologies
James H. Shore, Editor

RECENT ISSUES

December 2018
Sexual and Gender Identity Disorders
Charles Freeman and Kenneth R. Zucker,
Editors

September 2018
Neuromodulation
Noah S. Philip, Editors

June 2018
Psychodynamic Psychiatry
Thomas N. Franklin, Editor

SERIES OF RELATED INTEREST

Child and Adolescent Psychiatric Clinics of North America
Available at: www.childpsych.theclinics.com

THE CLINICS ARE AVAILABLE ONLINE!
Access your subscription at:
www.theclinics.com

Preface

Eating Disorders 2018: New Insights in Diagnosis, Research, and Treatment

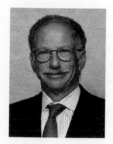
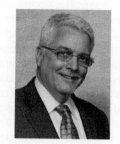

Harry A. Brandt, MD   Steven F. Crawford, MD
Editors

Eating disorders stand out as particularly complex multifaceted psychiatric illnesses with extreme morbidity and mortality. In the United States, conservative estimates suggest that 30 million people struggle with eating disorders, with high rates of medical complications and the highest suicide rate of all psychiatric diagnoses. Commonly with onset early in life, many patients do not achieve their fullest potential. Despite the human suffering, and significant family, social, and economic burden of these conditions, research funding, understanding of causes, and new treatment development have all lagged behind many other psychiatric and nonpsychiatric illnesses of comparable incidence and severity, such as schizophrenia or juvenile onset diabetes. Fortunately, this is finally changing. While we were very pleased to be asked by Dr Trivedi to undertake the role of guest editors to assemble a group of leading international experts to provide a comprehensive update on eating disorders, we were also aware of the daunting challenge that this would pose. There have been so many exciting developments in the past several years; it was difficult to choose what to include. Since eating disorders are often unrecognized, and in many cases, left untreated, we viewed this as a welcomed opportunity for leading experts to update both psychiatric and nonpsychiatric clinicians in this area of critical need. As we began to plan our approach and were feeling a bit overwhelmed with the magnitude of our task, the editors of the *Psychiatric Clinics of North America* graciously agreed to allow us to split our work into two issues. Part 1 focuses on the evolution of diagnostic

Psychiatr Clin N Am 42 (2019) xiii–xv
https://doi.org/10.1016/j.psc.2018.11.001
0193-953X/19/© 2018 Published by Elsevier Inc.

psych.theclinics.com

classification and current research, while part 2 will examine new developments in clinical treatment.

Part 1 begins with an article by Dr Walsh, who is a leading authority on diagnosis and who chairs the Eating Disorders Workgroup for *Diagnostic and Statistical Manual of Mental Disorders, Fifth Edition* (*DSM-5*). He gives a historical overview of eating disorder nomenclature, implications of the most recent changes in diagnostic criteria, and what we might expect going forward. Drs Kan and Treasure provide an overview of recent research on anorexia nervosa with a focus on individualized treatment elements targeting starvation and social exclusion as powerful perpetuating factors in chronic illness. The contributions of Dr Treasure's group have been immense, including promotion of a collaborative care model in the treatment of eating disorders. Dr Wade, a renown clinical and research leader, presents an update on current issues in the diagnosis and treatment of bulimia nervosa highlighting the significant impairments seen in the physical and emotional health of patients as well as strategies to effectively engage and treat patients. We were pleased that Dr Hilbert agreed to address recent research on binge-eating disorder, emphasizing in her excellent review that the illness is underdiagnosed and often ineffectively treated despite available evidence-based treatments and potentially efficacious pharmacologic intervention. Drs Katzman, Norris, and Zucker give a comprehensive overview of current knowledge of avoidant restrictive food intake disorder, which is newly classified in *DSM-5*. Drs Bulik, Blake, and Austin present a concise and cogent summary for clinicians of the emerging genetic understanding of the eating disorders. Dr Bulik's group has remained on the forefront of elucidation of the genetic underpinnings of the eating disorders for decades. Drs Steinglass, Berner, and Attia, from two of the most long-standing and established clinical research programs at Columbia and University of California, San Diego, give us an intriguing overview of application of cognitive neuroscience for understanding the chronic maladaptive behaviors in eating disorders with important implication for current understanding and future treatment of these disorders. Dr Seitz, Trinh, and Herpertz-Dahlmann provide a timely and important overview of the microbiome and its potential implications for starvation, refeeding, and possible new treatments. Drs Wagner and Vitousek propose an intriguing method to classify individuals with eating disorders by temperament and personality features as opposed to diagnostic criteria in order to better understand cause and develop effective treatment models. Dr Weissman cogently reviews the complex area of risk factors/sociocultural influences in the development of eating disorders. Drs McLean and Paxton then provide an intriguing review and discussion on the role of body image and body dissatisfaction in the development and perpetuation of eating disorders. Finally, Dr Bryant-Waugh presents a broad overview of some of the unique issues and challenges faced in treating eating disorders in children.

We are very thankful for each of these authors, all of whom are esteemed leaders in our field, for their gracious willingness to share their expertise and experience with all of us. We learned much as we read these articles, and we are confident that readers will find them compelling and important. We would also like to thank Dr Trivedi for the opportuntiy to edit these issues for the *Psychiatric Clinics of North America*. It is our hope that this update on eating disorders will be of great value to both the eating disorder specialist and the generalist, all clinicians working daily in the trenches, in their effort to ease the burden of these difficult but treatable illnesses.

Harry A. Brandt, MD
Center for Eating Disorders at
Sheppard Pratt
Department of Psychiatry
University of Maryland
St. Joseph Medical Center
Physician Pavilion North, Suite 300
6535 North Charles Street
Towson, MD 21204, USA

Steven F. Crawford, MD
Center for Eating Disorders at
Sheppard Pratt
University of Maryland
St. Joseph Medical Center
Physician Pavilion North, Suite 300
6535 North Charles Street
Towson, MD 21204, USA

E-mail addresses:
harry@brandtmd.com (H.A. Brandt)
scrawford@sheppardpratt.org (S.F. Crawford)

Eating Disorders Overview of Diagnostic Considerations

Diagnostic Categories for Eating Disorders
Current Status and What Lies Ahead

B. Timothy Walsh, MD

KEYWORDS

- *DSM-5* • Eating disorders • Anorexia nervosa • Bulimia nervosa
- Binge-eating disorder • ARFID

KEY POINTS

- Binge-eating disorder was officially recognized in *Diagnostic and Statistical Manual of Mental Disorders* (*DSM-5*).
- Criteria for avoidant/restrictive food intake disorder, a pattern of persistent restrictive eating, were articulated for the first time in *DSM-5*.
- *DSM-5* introduced severity ratings for anorexia nervosa, bulimia nervosa, and binge-eating disorder.

INTRODUCTION

The publication of the *Diagnostic and Statistical Manual of Mental Disorders* (Third Edition) (*DSM-III*) by the American Psychiatric Association (APA) in 1980 was a landmark event in the nosology of mental disorders and laid the foundation for the current definitions of most mental illnesses, including the eating disorders. *DSM-III* provided diagnostic criteria for anorexia nervosa and bulimia. *DSM-III-R* tweaked these criteria slightly and added "nervosa" to the title of bulimia. *DSM-IV* likewise made minor adjustments to the criteria for these 2 disorders but, more significantly, provided, in an appendix, suggested criteria for the diagnosis of binge-eating disorder. *DSM-5* was published in 2013, almost 20 years after *DSM-IV*, and introduced several significant changes. The criteria for anorexia nervosa and bulimia nervosa were again altered slightly, but, more importantly, binge-eating disorder was officially recognized. In addition, in *DSM-5*, the *DSM-IV* section entitled "Disorders Usually First Diagnosed in Infancy, Childhood, or Adolescence" was eliminated, reflecting the fact that almost all psychiatric disorders begin early in life. As a result, 3 disorders, pica, rumination,

Disclosures: Dr B.T. Walsh has received royalties from McGraw-Hill, UpToDate, Guilford Press, and Oxford University Press.
New York State Psychiatric Institute, Columbia University Medical Center, 1051 Riverside Drive, New York, NY 10032, USA
E-mail address: btw1@cumc.columbia.edu

Psychiatr Clin N Am 42 (2019) 1–10
https://doi.org/10.1016/j.psc.2018.10.001
0193-953X/19/© 2018 Elsevier Inc. All rights reserved.

and feeding disorder of infancy or early childhood, were added to the eating disorders section, which was retitled "Feeding and Eating Disorders." Finally, as discussed later, feeding disorder of infancy or early childhood was expanded and renamed avoidant/restrictive food intake disorder (ARFID).

This article highlights important features of the current *DSM-5* criteria for feeding in Eating Disorders and discusses challenges and future directions.

ANOREXIA NERVOSA

There is a broad and long-standing consensus regarding the essential features of anorexia nervosa: a relentless pursuit of thinness leading to an abnormally low body weight accompanied by a profound distortion of body image. *DSM-5* attempts to capture these features efficiently via 3 criteria (**Box 1**). Criterion A calls for "restriction of energy intake," implying that the caloric restriction is voluntary, "leading to a significantly low body weight." One of the small but significant changes from *DSM-IV* in this criterion was the elimination of the parenthetic phrase that contained the numerical guideline "body weight less than 85% of that expected." Even though provided only as an example, this phrase was the source of significant confusion both because it was sometimes interpreted as a specific, required threshold and because it was unclear how to determine what weight was "expected." During the development of *DSM-5*, some researchers suggested that the addition of a specific guideline, such as a body mass index (BMI) less than 18.5 kg/m^2 for adults, would enhance the reliability of this criterion. This perspective had validity, but, in the end, because the primary purpose of *DSM-5* is to provide guidance for clinicians, it was decided to allow for the exercise of clinical judgment and therefore not to include any numerical suggestions in criterion A. However, the text of *DSM-5* provides extensive information to assist the clinician in deciding of whether an individual's weight is "significantly low" by referencing several widely used guidelines.

The most substantial change in the criteria for anorexia nervosa from *DSM-IV* was the elimination of the criterion requiring amenorrhea. There were 2 reasons for this change. First, there were several exceptions to its use in *DSM-IV*: men, prepubertal and postmenopausal women, and women on oral contraceptives were all exempt from the requirement for amenorrhea. Second, a literature review documented several publications describing women who met all the criteria for anorexia nervosa but reported some spontaneous menstrual activity.[1] The text for *DSM-5* emphasizes that

---

Box 1
Diagnostic and Statistical Manual of Mental Disorders-5 criteria for anorexia nervosa

A. Restriction of energy intake relative to requirements leading to a significantly low body weight in the context of age, sex, developmental trajectory, and physical health. Significantly low weight is defined as a weight that is less than minimally normal, or, for children and adolescents, less than that minimally expected.

B. Intense fear of gaining weight or becoming fat, or persistent behavior that interferes with weight gain, even though at a significantly low weight.

C. Disturbance in the way in which one's body weight or shape is experienced, undue influence of body shape or weight on self-evaluation, or persistent lack of recognition of the seriousness of current low body weight.

Reprinted from the Diagnostic and statistical manual of mental disorders. 5th edition. (Copyright ©2013). American Psychiatric Association. All Rights Reserved; with permission.

amenorrhea is a commonly associated feature of anorexia nervosa, as are several other physiologic abnormalities.

DSM-5 retained the subtyping scheme for anorexia nervosa introduced in *DSM-IV*, whereby individuals are classified as having either the binge-eating/purging type if they engage in recurrent episodes of binge eating or purging or the restricting type if they do not. Individuals with the binge-eating/purging type are at greater risk for fluid and electrolyte disturbances and are more likely to engage in other impulsive behaviors compared with those with the restricting type.

BULIMIA NERVOSA

The *DSM-5* criteria for bulimia nervosa (**Box 2**) differ in only minor ways from those published in *DSM-III-R* in 1987. The key requirements are recurrent episodes of binge eating followed by inappropriate behaviors aimed to avoid weight gain, such as self-induced vomiting. An episode of binge eating is characterized by the consumption of an unusually large amount of food and a sense of loss of control over eating behavior during the eating episode. In addition, the individual experiences an inordinate concern over body weight and shape.

A persistent problem with the criteria for bulimia nervosa (and for binge-eating disorder) is what precisely constitutes an unusually large amount of food, which is defined as "an amount of food that is definitely larger than what most individuals would eat in a similar period of time under similar circumstances." Suggestions have been made to use a specific number of calories, such as 1000 Kcal, as a threshold, but have never been widely adopted. Guidance regarding the Eating Disorder Examination, a semi-structured interview widely used in research settings, includes specific quantities of food items that interviewers can use to aid their assessments, and well-trained interviewers attain substantial reproducibility in what constitutes a binge. Nonetheless, the requirement for clinical judgments that, in the end, are at least somewhat arbitrary is problematic.

The *DSM-5* criteria for bulimia nervosa differ in 2 small ways from those in *DSM-IV*. First, the required average minimum frequency of binge eating over the prior 3 months (criterion C) was reduced from 2 episodes to one per week. This change was based on research documenting the existence of individuals who engaged in binge eating at this relatively low frequency.[2] Second, a subtyping scheme introduced in *DSM-IV* that classed individuals as having either the purging or the nonpurging subtype was

---

Box 2
Diagnostic and Statistical Manual of Mental Disorders-5 criteria for bulimia nervosa

A. Recurrent episodes of binge eating.

B. Recurrent inappropriate compensatory behavior to prevent weight gain, such as self-induced vomiting; misuse of laxatives, diuretics, or other medications; fasting; or excessive exercise.

C. The binge eating and inappropriate behavior both occur, on average, at least once a week for 3 months.

D. Self-evaluation is unduly influenced by body shape and weight.

E. The disturbance does not occur exclusively during episodes of anorexia nervosa.

Reprinted from the Diagnostic and statistical manual of mental disorders. 5th edition. (Copyright ©2013). American Psychiatric Association. All Rights Reserved; with permission.

eliminated. Very little information is available in the published literature on the similarities and differences of individuals with these subtypes, and most reports focus on individuals who engage in self-induced vomiting after binge eating.

BINGE-EATING DISORDER

As noted in the introduction, tentative criteria for the diagnosis of binge-eating disorder were included in an appendix of *DSM-IV*. In the almost 2 decades that elapsed between *DSM-IV* and *DSM-5*, a very large body of literature emerged describing the characteristics of individuals with binge-eating disorder and the efficacy of a range of psychological and pharmacologic treatments. This accumulated knowledge provided the foundation for the official recognition of binge-eating disorder in *DSM-5*. Remarkably, only a slight change was made to the criteria provided in the *DSM-IV* appendix.

The criteria for binge-eating disorder (**Box 3**) strongly resemble those for bulimia nervosa. Criterion A requires recurrent episodes of binge eating, using the identical criteria used in bulimia nervosa. Criterion B describes markers indicative of a sense of loss of control, such as eating rapidly and eating alone out of embarrassment, and criterion C requires that the individual experiences marked distress over the binge eating. The only change made in the criteria proposed in *DSM-IV* was in criterion D, which describes the required minimum frequency of binge eating. In *DSM-IV*, the average minimum occurrence was episodes of binge eating occurring on 2 *days* per week over the prior 6 months; in *DSM-5*, this was changed to an average minimum of one *episode* of binge eating per week over the past 3 months, parallel to criterion C for bulimia nervosa.

AVOIDANT/RESTRICTIVE FOOD INTAKE DISORDER

One of the most important developments in *DSM-5* related to eating disorders was the articulation of criteria for ARFID. When it became clear that the disorders in the feeding disorder section of *DSM-IV* were to be combined with those in the eating disorders section, the Eating Disorders Work Group reviewed the state of knowledge and utility

---

Box 3
Diagnostic and Statistical Manual of Mental Disorders-5 criteria for binge-eating disorder

A. Recurrent episodes of binge eating.

B. The binge-eating episodes are associated with 3 (or more) of the following:
   1. Eating much more rapidly than normal.
   2. Eating until feeling uncomfortably full.
   3. Eating large amounts of food when not feeling physically hungry.
   4. Eating alone because of being embarrassed by how much one is eating.
   5. Feeling disgusted with oneself, depressed, or very guilty after overeating.

C. Marked distress regarding binge eating is present.

D. The binge eating occurs, on average, at least once a week for 3 months.

E. The binge eating is not associated with the recurrent use of inappropriate compensatory behavior as in bulimia nervosa and does not occur exclusively during the course of bulimia nervosa or anorexia nervosa.

Reprinted from the Diagnostic and statistical manual of mental disorders. 5th edition. (Copyright ©2013). American Psychiatric Association. All Rights Reserved; with permission.

Box 4
Diagnostic and Statistical Manual of Mental Disorders-5 criteria for avoidant/restrictive food intake disorder

A. An eating or feeding disturbance (eg, apparent lack of interest in eating or food; avoidance based on the sensory characteristics of food; concern about aversive consequences of eating) as manifested by persistent failure to meet appropriate nutritional and/or energy needs leading to one or more of the following:
   1. Significant weight loss (or failure to gain weight or faltering growth in children).
   2. Significant nutritional deficiency.
   3. Dependence on enteral feeding or oral nutritional supplements.
   4. Marked interference with psychosocial functioning.

B. The disturbance is not better explained by lack of available food or an associated culturally sanctioned practice.

C. The eating disturbance does not occur exclusively during the course of anorexia nervosa or bulimia nervosa, and there is no evidence of a disturbance in the way in which one's body weight or shape is experienced.

D. The eating disorder is not attributable to a concurrent medical condition or not better explained by another mental disorder. If the eating disturbance occurs in the context of another condition or disorder, the severity of the eating disturbance exceeds that routinely associated with the condition or disorder and warrants additional clinical attention.

Reprinted from the Diagnostic and statistical manual of mental disorders. 5th edition. (Copyright ©2013). American Psychiatric Association. All Rights Reserved; with permission.

---

of the feeding disorders.[3] The category feeding disorder of infancy or early childhood was introduced in *DSM-IV* to describe individuals less than 6 years old who had failed to gain or lost weight not due to a general medical condition such as esophageal reflux. A search of the literature published since *DSM-IV* revealed virtually no articles referring to this diagnosis, and it appeared to be little used in clinical practice. On the other hand, the Work Group became aware that a significant number of individuals, many but not all children and adolescents, were presenting for clinical treatment because of restrictive eating behavior that was not associated with the overconcern with shape and weight and other psychological characteristics of individuals with anorexia nervosa. For example, a youngster might have a nasty bout of vomiting after a meal due to a viral infection, and subsequently avoid eating solid food out of a fear of more vomiting.

These considerations led to the development of criteria for ARFID (**Box 4**). Criterion A describes the salient behavioral feature, an eating disturbance leading to inadequate intake of a normal range of foods and resulting in weight loss, a nutritional deficiency, dependence on nutritional supplements, and/or marked interference with psychosocial functioning.[a] Criteria B, C, and D serve to exclude individuals with restrictive food intake due to another psychiatric disorder, such as anorexia nervosa, to a general medical condition, or to the lack of available food or a practice sanctioned by the individual's culture. These criteria aimed to include individuals who met criteria for the *DSM-IV* Feeding Disorder of Infancy or Early Childhood but also individuals with a

---

[a] As this article goes to press, the APA is considering a change to criterion A for ARFID to eliminate some ambiguity in this criterion. The stem of criterion A includes the clause, "as manifested by persistent failure to meet appropriate nutritional and/or energy needs;" however, criterion A.4 does not describe a manifestation of a nutritional problem. To address this issue, it has been proposed to delete the clause in the stem, so that marked psychosocial impairment alone would clearly satisfy criterion A.

much broader range of presentations. Therefore, the individuals meeting criteria for ARFID comprise a heterogeneous group.

Many young individuals with ARFID present to pediatricians or adolescent medicine specialists, and early studies from such clinicians provided preliminary information regarding the frequency and characteristics of individuals meeting criteria for ARFID[4,5]; such data were instrumental in persuading the *DSM-5* Task Force to approve the inclusion of ARFID. Although it will take some time to characterize the clinical features and course of individuals with ARFID in detail, and to determine if there are distinct subgroups within this broad category, significant work is underway. At the time this article was written in mid-2018, a PubMed search of "ARFID" since 2013 yielded 56 "hits," documenting substantial interest in the investigation of this disorder.

PICA AND RUMINATION DISORDER

Pica (**Box 5**) and rumination disorder (**Box 6**) have been included in the *DSM* since *DSM-III* and remain in *DSM-5*. The only changes from *DSM-IV* were minor clarifications of wording and noting in the text that these disorders may develop in adults as well as in infants and children.

OTHER SPECIFIED FEEDING OR EATING DISORDER

Individuals with a clinically significant disturbance of eating behavior the symptoms of which do not fulfill the criteria for any of the 6 disorders described previously can be described as having another "specified feeding or eating disorder," a category equivalent to an eating disorder not otherwise specified in *DSM-IV*. *DSM-5* includes very brief descriptions of 5 presentations that have been recognized clinically but about which there is insufficient knowledge to justify formal recognition.

DIAGNOSTIC HIERARCHY

Implicit in the *DSM-5* criteria for feeding and eating disorders is a diagnostic hierarchy. Criterion E of bulimia nervosa indicates that this disorder cannot be used to describe individuals who also meet criteria for anorexia nervosa; such individuals should be classified as having the binge-eating/purging subtype of anorexia nervosa. Similarly, criterion E for binge-eating disorder prohibits assignment of this disorder to individuals

---

Box 5
Diagnostic and Statistical Manual of Mental Disorders-5 criteria for pica

A. Persistent eating of nonnutritive, nonfood substances over a period of at least 1 month.

B. The eating of nonnutritive, nonfood substances is inappropriate to the developmental level of the individual.

C. The eating behavior is not part of a culturally supported or socially normative practice.

D. If the eating behavior occurs in the context of another mental disorder (e.g., intellectual disability [intellectual developmental disorder], autism spectrum disorder, schizophrenia) or medical condition (including pregnancy), it is sufficiently severe to warrant additional clinical attention.

Reprinted from the Diagnostic and statistical manual of mental disorders. 5th edition. (Copyright ©2013). American Psychiatric Association. All Rights Reserved; with permission.

> **Box 6**
> *Diagnostic and Statistical Manual of Mental Disorders-5* criteria for rumination disorder
>
> A. Repeated regurgitation of food over a period of at least 1 month. Regurgitated food may be rechewed, reswallowed, or spit out.
>
> B. The repeated regurgitation is not attributable to an associated gastrointestinal or other medical condition (eg, gastroesophageal reflux, pyloric stenosis).
>
> C. The eating disturbance does not occur exclusively during the course of anorexia nervosa, bulimia nervosa, binge-eating disorder, or avoidant/restrictive food intake disorder.
>
> D. If the symptoms occur in the context of another mental disorder (eg, intellectual disability [intellectual developmental disorder] or another neurodevelopmental disorder), they are sufficiently severe to warrant additional clinical attention.
>
> *Reprinted from* the Diagnostic and statistical manual of mental disorders. 5th edition. (Copyright ©2013). American Psychiatric Association. All Rights Reserved; with permission.

who meet criteria for anorexia nervosa or bulimia nervosa. In this fashion, the diagnostic criteria for anorexia nervosa, bulimia nervosa, binge-eating disorder, and rumination disorder are mutually exclusive. Criterion C for ARFID excludes the simultaneous diagnosis of either anorexia nervosa or bulimia nervosa, but is silent regarding binge-eating disorder. Therefore, *DSM-5* does not explicitly exclude describing an individual as having ARFID and binge-eating disorder simultaneously. However, given that the former is characterized by restrictive eating and the latter by binge eating, such a scenario is presumably rare. Finally, it should be noted that a diagnosis of pica can be assigned simultaneously with any other feeding or eating disorder.

SEVERITY RATINGS

In an attempt to aid clinical management, *DSM-5* included severity ratings for several disorders, including anorexia nervosa, bulimia nervosa, and binge-eating disorder. For each disorder, the minimum severity rating is based primarily on the level of a key diagnostic element: for anorexia nervosa, current BMI; for bulimia nervosa, the frequency of inappropriate compensatory behavior; and, for binge-eating disorder, the frequency of binge eating. The severity rating may be increased beyond the minimum to reflect other symptoms.

Because the medical complications of anorexia nervosa are closely related to weight loss and because lower BMI has been linked to poor outcome and mortality,[6] basing the rating of current severity for an individual with anorexia nervosa on this factor seems appropriate. Linking the severity ratings of bulimia nervosa and binge-eating disorder to the frequencies of purging and binge eating, respectively, is not unreasonable, but it is not as clear that these behavioral features are closely associated with acute complications and longer-term outcome. Several studies have begun to explore the degree to which the *DSM-5* severity ratings are related to psychopathologic measures and outcome. Some,[7–11] but not all,[12–15] have suggested the severity ratings have merit. Substantial additional work is needed to assess the value of these ratings in clinical management and how the ratings might be improved. In particular, because the rationale for the ratings in *DSM-5* is to provide assistance with clinical management, it would be important to know to what degree the current rating of severity is linked to an individual's need for a higher level of acute care, and whether the rating of severity improves with treatment of known efficacy.

EPIDEMIOLOGY

For several reasons, it is important to assess the impact of changes introduced in *DSM-5* on the epidemiology of eating disorders. One of the major problems with the criteria in *DSM-IV* was that a substantial fraction of individuals presenting for treatment of an eating disorder did not meet criteria for either anorexia nervosa or bulimia nervosa, the only 2 formally defined eating disorders in *DSM-IV*, and therefore received the nonspecific diagnosis, eating disorder not otherwise classified. Evidence from a modest number of studies published since the introduction of *DSM-5* provides evidence that the changes introduced in *DSM-5* have led to a reduction in the use of the nonspecific category.[16]

In addition, concerns were raised during the development of *DSM-5* that the official recognition of binge-eating disorder was an example of pathologizing normality and would lead to inappropriately inflated prevalence estimates. A recent study examined the 12-month and lifetime prevalence of anorexia nervosa, bulimia nervosa, and binge-eating disorder according to *DSM-5* criteria in a very large (36,306 participants) survey of US adults.[17] The estimates of 12-month prevalence were surprisingly low, less than 1% for each of the disorders. Such data, which are broadly consistent with prior studies, indicate that, when rigorously applied, the *DSM-5* criteria for eating disorders do not yield population frequencies that seem unreasonable or suggest that a commonly occurring pattern of normal behavior is being characterized as pathologic.

INTERNATIONAL CLASSIFICATION OF DISEASES

By treaty, the United States is required to use the *International Classification of Diseases (ICD)* published by the World Health Organization to tabulate the frequency of disorders, including mental disorders. In order to provide more specificity for clinical use, the National Center for Health Statistics has developed a "clinical modification" of the *ICD (ICD-CM)*; it is that version which clinicians are required to use to describe the diagnoses of individuals admitted to hospitals and to request payment from medical insurance programs and Medicare. In October, 2015, the United States adopted the use of *ICD-10-CM*, and *DSM-5* provides these codes (eg, F50.2 for bulimia nervosa) in several locations. *ICD-10* was actually published in the early 1990s, and there are serious limitations on how well it maps on to *DSM-5*. For example, although there is a code for binge-eating disorder in *ICD-10-CM*, there is no description of that disorder in the *ICD-10*.

The development of *ICD-11* has been completed, and extensive efforts have been made to align *ICD-11* with *DSM-5*. The current draft of *ICD-11* has the same 6 formally defined feeding and eating disorders as does *DSM-5*, and the descriptions of the key features of each disorder are extremely similar.[18] One potentially problematic difference is that the definition of an episode of binge eating in the description of bulimia nervosa and of binge-eating disorder in *ICD-11* does not explicitly require the consumption of an abnormally large amount of food. Therefore, it is possible that an individual who frequently induces vomiting after experiencing a subjective sense of loss of control while eating only modest amounts of food might be assigned a diagnosis of bulimia nervosa according to *ICD-11* but not according to the *DSM-5* criteria. However, the expectation is that there will be a high degree of concordance between these 2 prominent diagnostic systems.

It should be noted that it is not clear when the United States will adopt the *ICD-11* coding scheme. Given that *ICD-10-CM* was only adopted in 2015 (more than 20 years after *ICD-10* was published by World Health Organization), it is likely to be many years until *ICD-11* is used in the United States.

LOOKING AHEAD

The formal classification of feeding and eating disorders, as articulated in *DSM-5* and *ICD-11*, is broadly accepted and has clinical utility. However, there are several important issues that it is hoped future study will address. For example, there is an obvious need for clarification of the characteristics and possible subgroups of ARFID. The validity and utility of the severity specifiers introduced in *DSM-5* require additional study and possible modification. To facilitate the continuous incorporation of important new findings that may emerge on these and other topics, the APA has made a major change in the way proposed modifications to the *DSM* criteria and text will be reviewed and implemented. All previous revisions to *DSM* criteria were made en masse. After a variable number of years had passed after the publication of an edition, a Task Force and multiple Work Groups were assembled to review the entirety of the *DSM* and make recommendations for change. This process was administratively cumbersome, slow, and expensive, and excluded the possibility of making modest but useful changes in the criteria for single disorders before a review and possible revision of criteria for all disorders. The APA is now considering changes to *DSM-5* on a rolling basis and permits anyone to submit a proposal for change. Details regarding the requirements for making submissions and the mechanisms by which they will be reviewed are described at www.dsm5.org.

Future research needs to address broader problems, as well. Although *DSM*, like the *ICD*, is a categorical system, many of the clinical phenomena that these systems attempt to capture exist along a spectrum, and, inevitably, there is some degree of arbitrariness in where the boundaries between disorders are drawn. The severity specifiers in *DSM-5* are a first attempt to add continuous information to a categorical system, but it is clear additional work is needed. Finally, as is widely recognized, although the *DSM-5* is clearly useful to clinicians, the categories are not based on knowledge of underlying psychobiological disturbances. A simple illustration of this fact is that there is virtually no way to confirm the accuracy of a clinician's assignment of a *DSM-5* diagnosis via an objective measure, such as a laboratory test. This significant limitation is a serious impediment to research on the origins of mental disorders and has led to the development of other noncategorical approaches to guide research, such as Research Domain Criteria.[19] However, given the challenges of such research and the complexity of mental illnesses, including the feeding and eating disorders, it seems likely that the *DSM* approach will remain in use for the foreseeable future.

ACKNOWLEDGMENT

The author wishes to thank Michael First MD for his useful comments regarding ICD.

REFERENCES

1. Attia E, Roberto CA. Should amenorrhea be a diagnostic criterion for anorexia nervosa? Int J Eat Disord 2009;42(7):581–9.
2. Wilson GT, Sysko R. Frequency of binge eating episodes in bulimia nervosa and binge eating disorder: Diagnostic considerations. Int J Eat Disord 2009;42(7): 603–10.
3. Bryant-Waugh R, Markham L, Kreipe RE, et al. Feeding and eating disorders in childhood. Int J Eat Disord 2010;43(2):98–111.
4. Fisher MM, Rosen DS, Ornstein RM, et al. Characteristics of avoidant/restrictive food intake disorder in children and adolescents: a "new disorder" in DSM-5. J Adolesc Health 2014;55(1):49–52.

5. Ornstein RM, Rosen DS, Mammel KA, et al. Distribution of eating disorders in children and adolescents using the proposed DSM-5 criteria for feeding and eating disorders. J Adolesc Health 2013;53(2):303–5.
6. Franko DL, Keshaviah A, Eddy KT, et al. A longitudinal investigation of mortality in anorexia nervosa and bulimia nervosa. Am J Psychiatry 2013;170(8):917–25.
7. Smink FR, van Hoeken D, Oldehinkel AJ, et al. Prevalence and severity of DSM-5 eating disorders in a community cohort of adolescents. Int J Eat Disord 2014; 47(6):610–9.
8. Grilo CM, Ivezaj V, White MA. Evaluation of the DSM-5 severity indicator for binge eating disorder in a clinical sample. Behav Res Ther 2015;71:110–4.
9. Grilo CM, Ivezaj V, White MA. Evaluation of the DSM-5 severity indicator for bulimia nervosa. Behav Res Ther 2015;67:41–4.
10. Grilo CM, Ivezaj V, White MA. Evaluation of the DSM-5 severity indicator for binge eating disorder in a community sample. Behav Res Ther 2015;66:72–6.
11. Gianini L, Roberto CA, Attia E, et al. Mild, moderate, meaningful? Examining the psychological and functioning correlates of DSM-5 eating disorder severity specifiers. Int J Eat Disord 2017;50(8):906–16.
12. Reas DL, Ro O. Investigating the DSM-5 severity specifiers based on thinness for adults with anorexia nervosa. Int J Eat Disord 2017;50(8):990–4.
13. Machado PP, Grilo CM, Crosby RD. Evaluation of the DSM-5 severity indicator for anorexia nervosa. Eur Eat Disord Rev 2017;25(3):221–3.
14. Dalle Grave R, Sartirana M, El Ghoch M, et al. DSM-5 severity specifiers for anorexia nervosa and treatment outcomes in adult females. Eat Behav 2018;31: 18–23.
15. Smith KE, Ellison JM, Crosby RD, et al. The validity of DSM-5 severity specifiers for anorexia nervosa, bulimia nervosa, and binge-eating disorder. Int J Eat Disord 2017;50(9):1109–13.
16. Lindvall Dahlgren C, Wisting L, Ro O. Feeding and eating disorders in the DSM-5 era: a systematic review of prevalence rates in non-clinical male and female samples. J Eat Disord 2017;5:56.
17. Udo T, Grilo CM. Prevalence and correlates of DSM-5-defined eating disorders in a nationally representative sample of U.S. adults. Biol Psychiatry 2018;84(5): 345–54.
18. Uher R, Rutter M. Classification of feeding and eating disorders: review of evidence and proposals for ICD-11. World Psychiatry 2012;11(2):80–92.
19. Cuthbert BN. Research domain criteria: toward future psychiatric nosologies. Dialogues Clin Neurosci 2015;17(1):89–97.

Recent Research and Personalized Treatment of Anorexia Nervosa

Carol Kan, MRCPsych, PhD[a],*, Janet Treasure, FRCPsych, FRCP, PhD[a,b]

KEYWORDS

- Anorexia nervosa • Staging • Personalized medicine • Social exclusion • Starvation

KEY POINTS

- Recent advances in understanding the multifactorial cause of anorexia nervosa are enhancing the way the illness is managed.
- Progress in neuropsychology is leading to a more individualized approach to treatment.
- Starvation and social exclusion are 2 key areas to target for successful treatment of anorexia nervosa.

INTRODUCTION

Anorexia nervosa is an illness with a high level of diversity because it includes physical and psychological elements, both of which contribute to the extreme disability and high mortality associated with the condition.[1] Anorexia nervosa often has an enduring course as illustrated by a recent study, which followed clinical cases presenting for treatment in the United States. At 9 years' follow-up, only 31% had recovered, although by 22 years follow-up, 63% had recovered.[2] When adopting a personalized approach to the management for anorexia nervosa, important questions for consideration are as follows:

- What is the level of risk?
- What is the form of the illness?

C. Kan is currently funded by the National Institute for Health Research (NIHR) and J. Treasure is partly funded by the NIHR Mental Health Biomedical Research Centre for Mental Health at South London and Maudsley National Health Service (NHS) Foundation Trust and King's College London.
[a] Section of Eating Disorders, Department of Psychological Medicine, Institute of Psychiatry, Psychology & Neuroscience, King's College London, 103, Denmark Hill, London SE5 8BP, UK;
[b] Eating Disorders Unit, South London and Maudsley NHS Foundation Trust, Monks Orchard Road, Beckenham BR3 3BX, UK
* Corresponding author.
E-mail address: carol.kan@kcl.ac.uk

- What potential resources from the individual's social structure and support network are available?

Clarifying answers to these questions will inform clinical judgment and decision making. Using knowledge from clinical trials and clinical experience as well as patient preferences,[3] the authors aim to develop an integrated personalized treatment plan that is both patient centered and evidence based.

WHAT IS THE LEVEL OF RISK?

Many factors can contribute to medical morbidity in anorexia nervosa, and establishing the level of risk to the patient is of paramount importance. Body mass index is a surrogate marker of risk and has now been introduced in classifying the severity of anorexia nervosa in the *Diagnostic and Statistical Manual of Mental Disorders* (fifth edition).[4] However, its utility is limited, and a multisystem evaluation of functioning can lead to a more precise risk assessment. In addition, physical health often interacts with aspects of psychological health, such as potential for self-harm, alcohol/substance abuse, binge eating, and purging behaviors. A thorough assessment of a broad range of risk factors should be considered in relation to elements such as motivation, resources, and social support. Higher-risk patients are often managed in hospital settings with inpatient or day-patient or partial hospitalization treatment programs, with some cases requiring treatment on an involuntary basis.

WHAT IS THE FORM OF THE ILLNESS? DEVELOPING A PERSONALIZED FORMULATION

Anorexia nervosa is a complex, multifactorial illness, spanning from childhood through adulthood. The adverse impact of starvation on the brain and the secondary physical and psychological problems resultant from protracted spans of untreated illness often interrupt normative adolescent developmental processes. It is therefore important to consider the timing of onset of illness. Important questions include the following:

- What is the duration of untreated illness?
- What is chronologic and developmental age of a patient?

Establishing a diagnostic formulation is an important step in developing a personalized management plan. It is helpful to consider the "3P's," namely predisposing, precipitating, and perpetuating factors. Genetic and neuropsychological elements described in other articles are also salient elements of a complete formulation (**Fig. 1**).

PREDISPOSING FACTORS

Table 1 summarizes some of the common predisposing factors seen in the development of anorexia nervosa. These studies must be interpreted in the context of low incidence rates of the illness,[40] because it limits the power of longitudinal studies in fully identifying significant predisposing factors. One way to circumvent this difficulty is to examine disordered eating, instead of full syndromal case status. In addition, larger studies of cases often require retrospective reporting, introducing potential recall bias. For the most part, where available, **Table 1** includes findings from case register studies, systematic reviews, or meta-analyses.

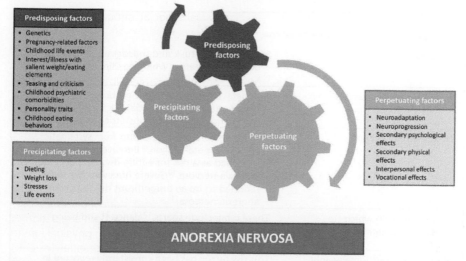

Fig. 1. The 3P's predisposing, precipitating, and perpetuating factors, of anorexia nervosa.

PRECIPITATING FACTORS

The most common pathway to the development of anorexia nervosa involves dieting and/or weight loss.[41] For most individuals, there is a deliberate strategy to lose weight or adopt "healthy" eating, although occasionally underlying medical illness may be the initial precipitant of disordered eating. In addition, reduction in caloric intake may occur in the context of life events and stressors.

PERPETUATING FACTORS

If anorexia nervosa remains untreated, its clinical signature becomes more severe over time. Therefore, it is essential that the understanding of perpetuating factors is improved, because they contribute to a protracted clinical course. In addition, these perpetuating factors can potentially be moderated and thus are useful targets of treatment. Several of the common perpetuating factors are summarized in **Table 2** and include neuroadaptation, neuroprogression, and social exclusion.[42,43] Neuroadaptation is a form of learning whereby addictive or avoidance behaviors become habitual (see Joanna E. Steinglass and colleagues' article, "Cognitive Neuroscience of Eating Disorders," in this issue). Prolonged starvation contributes to neuroprogressive deficits in brain structure and function.

Social cognition is another domain of vulnerability.[39] The reduced expression and interpretation of facial emotion during the acute phase of the illness contribute to interpersonal difficulties, which can in turn, impair vocational functioning. Moreover, people with anorexia nervosa have an increased sensitivity to threat[44] and negatively interpret social scenarios.[45] These clinical elements may be consequences of the state of high stress and arousal from the starvation state. Together, they are apt to impair social communication and reciprocity.

WHAT POTENTIAL RESOURCES FROM SOCIAL STRUCTURE AND SUPPORT ARE AVAILABLE?

The relevance of interpersonal functioning was poignantly and concisely highlighted in an article by a patient describing her journey through anorexia nervosa. She wrote that

Table 1 Predisposing factors of anorexia nervosa	
Genetics	See Cynthia M. Bulik and colleagues' article, "Eating Disorders Genetics: What the Clinician Needs to Know," in this issue
Pregnancy-related factors	Antenatal trauma[5,6] and low gestational age[7] have been suggested as potential risk factors. There is conflicting evidence for obstetric complications[8]
Childhood life events	There is no consistent reporting from systematic review or meta-analysis.[9] Bereavement has been identified as a risk for eating disorders but not for anorexia nervosa.[10] Severe life event has been reported to be an insignificant risk factor for anorexia nervosa[11]
Interest/illness in which weight and eating are salient	These can include sports,[12] dance,[13] and being diagnosed with type 1 diabetes[14,15]
Teasing/salience/stigma/weight labeling about weight, shape, and eating	This risk factor has been consistently reported in longitudinal studies,[16,17] systematic review, and meta-analysis[18]
Childhood eating behaviors	Both leanness and overweight during childhood have been identified as a predisposing factor in a longitudinal study,[19] in addition to childhood poor eating[20,21] and heightened appetite[22,23]
Childhood psychiatric comorbidities	Attention-deficit/hyperactivity disorder,[24] autism spectrum disorder,[25] anxiety,[26] and obsessive-compulsive disorders[27–29] have been noted
Personality traits	This includes rumination,[30] social anxiety,[31] attachment styles,[32] metacognition anomalies,[33] emotional regulation,[38] perfectionism,[34] social cognition,[39] emotional processing,[35,36] and self-esteem[37]

Whenever possible, citations include high-quality studies, systematic review, or meta-analysis.

"isolation" was one word that could encapsulate her experience.[46] The impairments in social cognition outlined above also contribute to the profound sense of isolation experienced by many patients with anorexia nervosa.

In addition, eating with others is a key element of social functioning, and taken together with the visible nature of the disorder, anorexia nervosa can have strong repercussions on close others. The starved state can elicit strong emotions of terror, horror, and even disgust in others, which is often combined with a protective response. Moreover, the resistance to the obvious simple solution "to eat" elicits frustration and hostility. These high levels of "expressed emotion" can serve to maintain or perpetuate the disorder.[47] Extremes of overprotection and hostility can also further perpetuate avoidance behavior, and families may gradually get drawn into accommodating or enabling the illness. These reactions also may occur with various staff members on inpatient/day-care units. A potential consequence of these various emotional reactions can be the developments of "splits" within the team and family. These fissures can lead to perpetuation of the disorder but also can cause relationship ruptures and dissipate the support structure.

Table 2	
Perpetuating factors of anorexia nervosa	
Neuroadaptation	Learning-dependent plasticity in which symptomatic behaviors become habitual, such as fears of food in anorexia nervosa
Neuroprogression	The secondary consequences of starvation on brain structure and function include reduced neuroplasticity. Complex cognitive functions, such as social cognition and integrative circuits, are also impaired
Secondary psychological effects	Many of the predisposing traits of rigidity, obsessive compulsive personality traits, anxiety, anhedonia, reduced social aptitude are accentuated by starvation
Secondary physical effects	The secondary physical consequences may be reinforcing for some individuals, such as secondary amenorrhea. For example, one theoretic explanation of anorexia nervosa considered that the psychosocial regression allowed avoidance of adult sexuality. For others, the overt signaling of "sickness/frailty" increases parental attachment behaviors and avoids the need to strive for adult autonomy
Interpersonal effects	Living with someone with an eating disorder can produce high levels of expressed emotion (overprotection, hostility and criticism). Family members over time accommodate to, or enable, the illness. These reactions can lead to tensions and fragmentation within the family and between the family and treatment team. Social isolation is a common consequence of the illness. Weight, shape, and diet can be of particular relevance in some families with eating disorders or metabolic anomalies
Vocational effects	Educational progress may be interrupted and there are often difficulties at work. Careers that have a focus on weight, shape, and eating may maintain the disorder

These factors are potential targets for change in treatment.

PLANNING TREATMENT

For the most part, people presenting to child and adolescent services are in the early stage of the illness, commonly with onset of 1 year or less. In contrast, people in later stages of illness are more likely to present to an adult service where many have had the illness for years, and some with recurring episodes. The type of treatment offered, such as the focus on the family in child and adolescent services, and the expected outcome, such as poorer response in the context of a prolonged illness in adults, is different between the services. However, regardless of context, a key for successful treatment lies in targeting starvation and social exclusion.

TARGETING STARVATION

Weight loss is a key perpetuating factor in anorexia nervosa, because the impact of starvation on both brain and body lead to consequences that serve in the longer term to exacerbate rather than resolve the stress and predisposing factors that may have triggered the illness. There are, however, many uncertainties about when, how, where, and with what help, weight can be restored and once restored, sustained.

An established and evidenced-based first-line treatment of adolescents is family-based treatment. Family-based treatment involves empowering parents to feed their children. The next level may include inpatient treatment, which is an effective method of restoring weight, but it can be followed by early relapse. In adolescents, a less-intensive, stepped-care approach with shorter inpatient stays and either day-care or task sharing with families appear to be a more cost-effective option.[48,49]

In adults, various forms of psychotherapy, including behavior change strategies to increase oral intake, have been developed and tested. They all produce similar effects: the proportion that recovers is small and weight restoration is poorly sustained.[50] To initiate and maintain weight restoration, fear of weight gain and the increasingly controlling and critical "anorexic voice" must be overcome. A personalized approach is essential to select the most appropriate treatment of an individual.

Promising, targeted approaches are also in development, for example, use of exposure to normal eating and challenging expectations to confront fears while learning new patterns of behavior by using habit-focused interventions are described elsewhere in this issue (see Joanna E. Steinglass and colleagues' article, "Cognitive Neuroscience of Eating Disorders," in this issue). It is possible that new neuromodulation and pharmacologic techniques may have a role in reversing some of the cascade of problems, such as reducing depressive symptoms, which can develop during the protracted course of starvation in anorexia nervosa.[51]

TARGETING SOCIAL EXCLUSION

Training carers with the skills to sidestep nonproductive interactions with patients is important, because it reduces carer distress and enhances patient well-being. Providing carers of inpatients with self-management tools can reduce carers' expressed emotion and distress,[52] therefore avoiding potential burnout. It also reduces readmission in the 6 months after discharge, whereas small improvements in both carers' behaviors and patients' symptoms were sustained 2 years later.[53] A similar pattern of improvements has also been noted by delivering this intervention to carers of adolescents receiving psychological therapy at outpatient units.[54]

SUMMARY

In conclusion, our field has come a long way from using treatments that are agnostic about cause. Newer developments in neuropsychology have allowed us to develop a better understanding of anorexia nervosa, and we are getting closer to adopting a personalized approach to treatment. Given the protracted course, any effort in reducing the devastating impact of the illness could improve the lives of people with anorexia nervosa and their families.

REFERENCES

1. Arcelus J, Mitchell AJ, Wales J, et al. Mortality rates in patients with anorexia nervosa and other eating disorders. A meta-analysis of 36 studies. Arch Gen Psychiatry 2011;68:724–31.

2. Eddy KT, Tabri N, Thomas JJ, et al. Recovery from anorexia nervosa and bulimia nervosa at 22-year follow-up. J Clin Psychiatry 2017;78(2):184–9.

3. Peterson CB, Becker CB, Treasure J, et al. The three-legged stool of evidence-based practice in eating disorder treatment: research, clinical, and patient perspectives. BMC Med 2016;14:69.

4. American Psychiatric Association. Diagnostic and statistical manual of mental disorders (DSM-5®). Washington, DC: American Psychiatric Pub; 2000.

5. Shoebridge P, Gowers SG. Parental high concern and adolescent-onset anorexia nervosa. A case-control study to investigate direction of causality. Br J Psychiatry 2000;176:132–7.
6. St-Hilaire A, Steiger H, Liu A, et al. A prospective study of effects of prenatal maternal stress on later eating-disorder manifestations in affected offspring: preliminary indications based on the Project Ice Storm cohort. Int J Eat Disord 2015; 48(5):512–6.
7. Goodman A, Heshmati A, Malki N, et al. Associations between birth characteristics and eating disorders across the life course: findings from 2 million males and females born in Sweden, 1975-1998. Am J Epidemiol 2014;179:852–63.
8. Krug I, Taborelli E, Sallis H, et al. A systematic review of obstetric complications as risk factors for eating disorder and a meta-analysis of delivery method and prematurity. Physiol Behav 2013;109:51–62.
9. Caslini M, Bartoli F, Crocamo C, et al. Disentangling the association between child abuse and eating disorders: a systematic review and meta-analysis. Psychosom Med 2016;78:79–90.
10. Su X, Liang H, Yuan W, et al. Prenatal and early life stress and risk of eating disorders in adolescent girls and young women. Eur Child Adolesc Psychiatry 2016; 25:1245–53.
11. Larsen JT, Munk-Olsen T, Bulik CM, et al. Early childhood adversities and risk of eating disorders in women: a Danish register-based cohort study. Int J Eat Disord 2017;50:1404–12.
12. Reardon CL, Factor RM. Sport psychiatry: a systematic review of diagnosis and medical treatment of mental illness in athletes. Sports Med 2010;40:961–80.
13. Hincapie CA, Cassidy JD. Disordered eating, menstrual disturbances, and low bone mineral density in dancers: a systematic review. Arch Phys Med Rehabil 2010;91:1777–89.e1.
14. De Paoli T, Rogers PJ. Disordered eating and insulin restriction in type 1 diabetes: a systematic review and testable model. Eat Disord 2018;26(4):343–60.
15. Toni G, Berioli MG, Cerquiglini L, et al. Eating disorders and disordered eating symptoms in adolescents with type 1 diabetes. Nutrients 2017;9(8) [pii:E906].
16. Haynos AF, Watts AW, Loth KA, et al. Factors predicting an escalation of restrictive eating during adolescence. J Adolesc Health 2016;59:391–6.
17. Puhl RM, Wall MM, Chen C, et al. Experiences of weight teasing in adolescence and weight-related outcomes in adulthood: a 15-year longitudinal study. Prev Med 2017;100:173–9.
18. Menzel JE, Schaefer LM, Burke NL, et al. Appearance-related teasing, body dissatisfaction, and disordered eating: a meta-analysis. Body Image 2010;7: 261–70.
19. Stice E, Gau JM, Rohde P, et al. Risk factors that predict future onset of each DSM-5 eating disorder: predictive specificity in high-risk adolescent females. J Abnorm Psychol 2017;126:38–51.
20. Karwautz A, Rabe-Hesketh S, Hu X, et al. Individual-specific risk factors for anorexia nervosa: a pilot study using a discordant sister-pair design. Psychol Med 2001;31:317–29.
21. Kotler LA, Cohen P, Davies M, et al. Longitudinal relationships between childhood, adolescent, and adult eating disorders. J Am Acad Child Adolesc Psychiatry 2001;40:1434–40.
22. Reed ZE, Micali N, Bulik CM, et al. Assessing the causal role of adiposity on disordered eating in childhood, adolescence, and adulthood: a Mendelian randomization analysis. Am J Clin Nutr 2017;106:764–72.

23. Sonneville KR, Calzo JP, Horton NJ, et al. Childhood hyperactivity/inattention and eating disturbances predict binge eating in adolescence. Psychol Med 2015;45:2511–20.

24. Nazar BP, Bernardes C, Peachey G, et al. The risk of eating disorders comorbid with attention-deficit/hyperactivity disorder: a systematic review and meta-analysis. Int J Eat Disord 2016;49(12):1045–57.

25. Westwood H, Eisler I, Mandy W, et al. Using the autism-spectrum quotient to measure autistic traits in anorexia nervosa: a systematic review and meta-analysis. J Autism Dev Disord 2016;46:964–77.

26. Meier SM, Bulik CM, Thornton LM, et al. Diagnosed Anxiety disorders and the risk of subsequent anorexia nervosa: a Danish population register study. Eur Eat Disord Rev 2015;23(6):524–30.

27. Anderluh MB, Tchanturia K, Rabe-Hesketh S, et al. Childhood obsessive-compulsive personality traits in adult women with eating disorders: defining a broader eating disorder phenotype. Am J Psychiatry 2003;160:242–7.

28. Degortes D, Zanetti T, Tenconi E, et al. Childhood obsessive-compulsive traits in anorexia nervosa patients, their unaffected sisters and healthy controls: a retrospective study. Eur Eat Disord Rev 2014;22:237–42.

29. Jacobi C, Hayward C, de Zwaan M, et al. Coming to terms with risk factors for eating disorders: application of risk terminology and suggestions for a general taxonomy. Psychol Bull 2004;130:19–65.

30. Smith KE, Mason TB, Lavender JM. Rumination and eating disorder psychopathology: a meta-analysis. Clin Psychol Rev 2018;61:9–23.

31. Kerr-Gaffney J, Harrison A, Tchanturia K. Social anxiety in the eating disorders: a systematic review and meta-analysis. Psychol Med 2018;48(15):2477–91.

32. Faber A, Dube L, Knauper B. Attachment and eating: a meta-analytic review of the relevance of attachment for unhealthy and healthy eating behaviors in the general population. Appetite 2018;123:410–38.

33. Sun X, Zhu C, So SHW. Dysfunctional metacognition across psychopathologies: a meta-analytic review. Eur Psychiatry 2017;45:139–53.

34. Limburg K, Watson HJ, Hagger MS, et al. The relationship between perfectionism and psychopathology: a meta-analysis. J Clin Psychol 2017;73:1301–26.

35. Oldershaw A, Hambrook D, Stahl D, et al. The socio-emotional processing stream in Anorexia Nervosa. Neurosci Biobehav Rev 2011;35:970–88.

36. Oldershaw A, Lavender T, Sallis H, et al. Emotion generation and regulation in anorexia nervosa: a systematic review and meta-analysis of self-report data. Clin Psychol Rev 2015;39:83–95.

37. Nicholls D, Statham R, Costa S, et al. Childhood risk factors for lifetime bulimic or compulsive eating by age 30 years in a British national birth cohort. Appetite 2016;105:266–73.

38. Aldao A, Nolen-Hoeksema S, Schweizer S. Emotion-regulation strategies across psychopathology: a meta-analytic review. Clin Psychol Rev 2010;30:217–37.

39. Caglar-Nazali HP, Corfield F, Cardi V, et al. A systematic review and meta-analysis of 'Systems for Social Processes' in eating disorders. Neurosci Biobehav Rev 2014;42:55–92.

40. Micali N, Hagberg KW, Petersen I, et al. The incidence of eating disorders in the UK in 2000-2009: findings from the General Practice Research Database. BMJ Open 2013;3(5). https://doi.org/10.1136/bmjopen-2013-002646.

41. Patton GC, Selzer R, Coffey C, et al. Onset of adolescent eating disorders: population based cohort study over 3 years. BMJ 1999;318(7186):765–8.

42. Treasure J, Russell G. The case for early intervention in anorexia nervosa: theoretical exploration of maintaining factors. Br J Psychiatry 2011;199:5–7.
43. Treasure J, Stein D, Maguire S. Has the time come for a staging model to map the course of eating disorders from high risk to severe enduring illness? An examination of the evidence. Early Interv Psychiatry 2014;9:173–84.
44. Harrison A, O'Brien N, Lopez C, et al. Sensitivity to reward and punishment in eating disorders. Psychiatry Res 2010;177(1–2):1–11.
45. Cardi V, Turton R, Schifano S, et al. Biased interpretation of ambiguous social scenarios in anorexia nervosa. Eur Eat Disord Rev 2017;25(1):60–4.
46. McKnight R, Boughton N. A patient's journey. Anorexia nervosa. BMJ 2009;339: b3800.
47. Treasure J, Nazar BP. Interventions for the carers of patients with eating disorders. Curr Psychiatry Rep 2016;18(2):16.
48. Herpertz-Dahlmann B, Schwarte R, Krei M, et al. Day-patient treatment after short inpatient care versus continued inpatient treatment in adolescents with anorexia nervosa (ANDI): a multicentre, randomised, open-label, non-inferiority trial. Lancet 2014;383:1222–9.
49. Madden S, Miskovic-Wheatley J, Wallis A, et al. A randomized controlled trial of in-patient treatment for anorexia nervosa in medically unstable adolescents. Psychol Med 2015;45(2):415–27.
50. Murray SB, Loeb KL, Le Grange D. Treatment outcome reporting in anorexia nervosa: time for a paradigm shift? J Eat Disord 2018;6:10.
51. Dalton B, Campbell IC, Schmidt U. Neuromodulation and neurofeedback treatments in eating disorders and obesity. Curr Opin Psychiatry 2017;30(6):458–73.
52. Hibbs R, Magill N, Goddard E, et al. Clinical effectiveness of a skills training intervention for caregivers in improving patient and caregiver health following inpatient treatment for severe anorexia nervosa: pragmatic randomised controlled trial. BJPsych Open 2015;1:56–66.
53. Magill N, Rhind C, Hibbs R, et al. Two-year follow-up of a pragmatic randomised controlled trial examining the effect of adding a carer's skill training intervention in inpatients with anorexia nervosa. Eur Eat Disord Rev 2016;24:122–30.
54. Hodsoll J, Rhind C, Micali N, et al. A pilot, multicentre pragmatic randomised trial to explore the impact of carer skills training on carer and patient behaviours: testing the cognitive interpersonal model in adolescent anorexia nervosa. Eur Eat Disord Rev 2017;25(6):551–61.

Recent Research on Bulimia Nervosa

Tracey D. Wade, PhD

KEYWORDS

• Bulimia nervosa • Assessment • Treatment • Epidemiology • Clinical features

KEY POINTS

• There has been a decrease in the presentation of bulimia nervosa (BN) in primary care but an increase in disordered eating not meeting full diagnostic criteria.
• Disordered eating is associated with long-term significant impairment to both physical and mental quality of life.
• BN is associated with a significantly higher likelihood of self-harm, suicide, and death.
• Assessment should adopt a motivationally enhancing stance given the high level of ambivalence associated with BN.
• Cognitive behavior therapy specific to eating disorders outperforms other active psychological comparisons.

DIAGNOSIS

Bulimia nervosa (BN) is an eating disorder that is characterized by 3 main diagnostic elements:

• Objective binge episodes (eating a large amount of food within a 2-hour period),
• Attempts to compensate for this binge eating (either through use of purging, driven exercise, fasting or underdosing with insulin in the presence of type I diabetes),
• Overevaluation of the importance of weight and/or shape.

Diagnostically, the required frequency of binge episodes and compensatory behaviors is once a week for a 3-month period.[1] In order to ascertain the presence or absence of some of these diagnostic criteria, definitions have typically been derived from the most frequently used assessment tool for eating disorders, the Eating Disorder Examination.[2] Fasting is defined as periods of 8 or more waking hours without eating anything to influence shape or weight. Driven exercise is defined as intensive

Disclosure Statement: No disclosures.
School of Psychology, Flinders University, GPO Box 2100, Adelaide, South Australia 5001, Australia
E-mail address: tracey.wade@flinders.edu.au

Psychiatr Clin N Am 42 (2019) 21–32
https://doi.org/10.1016/j.psc.2018.10.002

and vigorous physical activity associated with a compulsive quality, that is, having a strong negative reaction if prevented from exercising, interfering with day-to-day functioning by interrupting work or social commitments, and predominantly for the purpose of influencing weight or shape (and does not include competitive sport). During spans of disordered eating, at least moderate emphasis on the importance of weight and/or shape should be present (ie, overevaluation), such that it is considered to be an important influence on one's self-evaluation. BN is not given as a diagnosis if these behaviors occur during an episode of anorexia nervosa.

EPIDEMIOLOGY

Estimates of lifetime *Diagnostic and Statistical Manual of Mental Disorders* (Fourth Edition) *DSM-IV*[3] BN vary across studies, ranging from 1.5% to 4.6%. Estimates of lifetime *DSM-5*[1] BN, with more relaxed criteria, are between 4% and 6.7%.[4] Community incidence rates based on tracking eating disorders in general practice suggest that there has been a decrease in the presentation of BN in primary care across several countries.[5–7] There has, however, been an increase in disordered eating not necessarily meeting diagnostic criteria,[8] with 23% of women in community samples between 22 and 27 years reporting the presence of disordered eating (moderate dissatisfaction with weight or shape accompanied by either a body mass index <17.5, objective binge eating, self-induced vomiting, laxatives, diuretics, diet pills, or fasting) in the previous 12-month period.[9] It is worthy of note that such disordered eating is associated with long-term significant impairment to both physical and mental quality of life.[9]

CLINICAL FEATURES
Emergence

BN emerges somewhat later in life than anorexia nervosa, with binge and purge symptoms having a peak age of onset in late adolescence and early adulthood.[10,11] The mean age of emergence of BN is around 19 years of age, ranging from 10 to 29 years.[12] Around 24% to 31% of people with BN will have experienced a previous diagnosis of anorexia nervosa.[13]

Comorbidity

More than 70% of individuals with eating disorders report comorbidity,[14] with anxiety disorders (50%), mood disorders (40%), self-harm (20%), and substance use (10%) being the most common. All eating disorders are associated with a significantly higher likelihood of self-harm, suicide, and death,[15] with the standardized mortality ratios for suicide in BN around 7.5 per 100,000. Prevalence of nonfatal suicidal behavior (attempts and ideation) is also significantly elevated in BN, ranging from 15% to 40%.[16–19]

Emotion Regulation and Impulsivity

BN is associated with problems in emotional regulation. Compared with healthy controls, people with BN experience more difficulties with the following:

- Flexible use of adaptive and situationally appropriate strategies to modulate the duration and/or intensity of emotion,
- The ability to successfully inhibit impulsive behavior and maintain goal-directed behavior in the context of emotional distress,

- Awareness and acceptance of emotional states,
- A willingness to experience emotional distress in the pursuit of meaningful activities.[20]

Notable to BN and bulimic-spectrum disorder are significantly elevated levels of impulsivity when compared with control groups and those with restrictive disorders.[21] Of the various facets of impulsivity, sensation seeking or the tendency to pursue novel or exciting stimuli has the largest effect size association with bulimic symptoms.[22] In a sample of opposite sex twins, where the female twin had BN but the brother did not, there were shared risk factors between BN and generalized anxiety disorder, neuroticism, psychoactive substance use, and novelty seeking.[23] Numerous twin studies have examined comorbidity between bulimic disorders and substance use disorders (alcohol, illicit drug, and caffeine abuse/dependence), indicating the correlation between genetic risk factors is significant, ranging from 0.35 to 0.53,[24,25] with little overlap in environmental risk factors.

Neurobiological Disturbance

Emerging evidence suggests that neurobiological disturbances are also present in BN,[26] including high pain thresholds that persist after recovery, abnormal brain activation in response to tastes within brain regions typically involved in both interoceptive and taste processing, and disturbances in the insula that may impact multiple sensory domains. Dieting can lead to serotonin (5-HT) abnormalities, and some abnormalities in 5-HT function persist even after recovery.[27]

ASSESSMENT
Managing Ambivalence

Less than one-third of community cases with BN are detected by health professionals.[13] Several reasons account for this low rate, including the ambivalence and shame felt by patients, as outlined in **Table 1**. The ambivalence is driven largely by

Table 1
Why are so few cases of bulimia nervosa detected by health professionals?

Reasons	Evidence from the Literature
Ambivalence about the disorder and treatment; minimization of the consequences of disordered eating	Both men and women with high levels of eating disorder symptoms perceived BN as less serious and more acceptable than people with lower levels of symptoms[28,29]
Shame and stigma	Negative attitudes toward BN in terms of personal responsibility are shown by the community; men compared with women and lower education vs higher education predicted significantly higher stigmatizing attitudes[30]
Failure to ask	Patients (N = 260) consecutively referred and assessed for anxiety and depression and a specialist mental health outpatient service were assessed for disordered eating as part of their routine intake: 18.5% experienced eating problems, and 7.3% met criteria for an eating disorder[31]
Unfamiliarity with symptoms	A vignette study completed by 154 general practitioners gave a diagnosis of an eating disorder to <70% of cases with clear eating disorder presentation[32]

expectancies that thinness and control over weight, shape, and eating will lead to an improved life, including intrapersonal and interpersonal life functioning.[33,34] The assessment process shown in **Table 2** offers an important opportunity to explore the functions of the eating disorder, the fears of change, and concerns about self-efficacy, while also acquiring an understanding of the triggers and maintaining factors.[35] As such, it is useful to adopt a motivationally enhancing stance during assessment, conducting it in a manner consistent with the 5 key principles of motivational interviewing[36]:

- *Expressing empathy* reflects to the patient that ambivalence about change and treatment is normal and also takes care to avoid any suggestion of personal blame but normalizes the cycle of disordered eating driven by dietary restraint, binge eating, and attempts to compensate for the binge eating.
- *Developing discrepancy* recognizes that all patients have some concerns about what is occurring, and the assessment process tries to maximize the opportunity for the patient to verbalize concerns and reasons for change, known as "talking oneself into change."[37]
- *Avoiding argumentation* means that the assessor takes the stance of open and respectful curiosity, seeking to understand how the person got to this point. Complex reflections are helpful as part of this process, recognizing that, on the one hand, the patient is unsure about change, but on the other hand, feels that things cannot go on as they are.
- *Rolling with resistance* involves the recognition that assessment is an opportunity to invite new perspectives on the problem, but not impose them. As such, the patient is considered a partner in enquiry, figuring out whether their goals can be achieved in a way that does them less harm but is more likely to help them approach their goals in a manner that is consistent with their values.
- *Supporting self-efficacy* is of particular pertinence to BN given that confidence to effect personal change (self-efficacy) is a robust predictor of BN treatment outcome.[38] The patient may have arrived with well-meaning advice (from friends and professionals) to "just eat properly" or "just eat more," and clearly, if it was this simple, they would not be presenting for help. The compelling pull of the vicious cycle of disordered eating needs to be emphasized, while stressing the likelihood of significant improvement if the patient actively participates in an evidence-based therapy. This further involves a highlighting of the personal characteristics and strengths that the patient brings to therapy that suggests that they have the ability to change.

Depression, Suicidality, and Self-Harm

The assessment may highlight issues that require further attention before commencing therapy for BN, typically the presence of depression, self-harm, and suicidality. Although there is considerable evidence that antidepressants have some beneficial effect,[27] the most recent National Institute for Health and Care Excellence (NICE[39]) treatment guidelines recommend not offering medication as the sole treatment for BN, as relapse when medication is tapered is common, and evidence suggests no difference in outcome between psychotherapy and antidepressants at posttreatment.[40,41] Safety planning when self-harm and/or suicidality is present should be highly specific and operationalized. A link to one such plan is provided in **Table 2**. A comprehensive safety plan should be reviewed and updated regularly through the course of treatment.

Table 2
Unstructured assessment protocol for bulimia nervosa

Area	Specific Issues to Address
Understanding motivation for attendance	• Reason for attendance? Own concerns, other's concerns (who?), primary physician? • What troubles you the most about what is currently happening? • What would others who care about you (specify) be worried about?
Development of the eating disorder	• Developmental review of the eating disorder and accompanying weight history • Triggers for emergence of disordered eating (stressful life events, personality traits, dieting) • How did the disordered eating help you to cope?
Previous treatment experience	• Any previous treatment? • What did they do in treatment? • What was helpful or unhelpful?
Resultant impairment across the life domains	• What impact has disordered eating had on your life? • Address life domains: physical (ascertain presence of type 1 diabetes), psychological, family, work/education, friendships, getting on with life, social, romantic, being a good citizen, spiritual domains
Psychiatric comorbidity	• Other mental health issues, self and family? • Any accompanying treatment (including medication) • Indicators of impulsive behavior (shop lifting, drug & alcohol, unprotected sex) • Indicators of emotional regulation difficulty (self-cutting)
Maintaining factors	• Self-esteem and identity • Sense of effectiveness, achievement, and control • Perfectionism
Suicide risk	• Frequency and intensity of any thoughts, specificity of plans, previous attempts • https://www.beyondblue.org.au/get-support/beyondnow-suicide-safety-planning/create-beyondnow-safety-plan
Interpersonal functioning	• Who knows? • Who offers support? Who makes it worse? • Avoidance of social contact
Attitude toward therapy	Assess ambivalence, pros and cons, fears of change, possible benefits of change; use of 100-point Visual Analog Scales to assess importance of change, readiness to change, and self-efficacy (ie, confidence in one's ability to change). At this point, it may be useful to ask the patient permission to give them psycho-educational material to help them consider the costs and benefits more thoroughly
More detailed assessment of the disordered eating	Once rapport has been facilitated, more formalized assessment can be conducted with the following freely available diagnostic interviews or questionnaires: 1. Eating Disorder Examination: http://www.credo-oxford.com/pdfs/EDE_17.0D.pdf. 2. The Structured Inventory for Anorexic and Bulimic Eating Disorders (SIAB-EX): http://www.klinikum.uni-muenchen.de/Klinik-und-Poliklinik-fuer-Psychiatrie-und-Psychotherapie/de/forschung/forschungsfelder/essstoerungen/evaluation/index.html 3. The Eating Disorder Assessment for *DSM-5*: https://modeleda5.wordpress.com/

Medical Functioning

Assessment of medical functioning is essential across all eating disorders because weight-based markers alone do not suffice to indicate medical risk. There are specific areas of focus in the medical assessment for BN,[39] including but not limited to gastrointestinal disturbances, electrolyte abnormalities predisposing to cardiovascular issues, as well as the potential for permanent dental damage if self-induced vomiting is present. One vulnerable subgroup is patients with type 1 diabetes mellitus, where an increased prevalence of BN has been noted[42] that may be associated with insulin omission or underdosing. The presence of disordered eating leads to a 3-fold increase in the risk of retinopathy and microvascular complications.[43] Insulin omission appears to be most prevalent among young women aged between 15 and 30 years[44] and occurs in 34% of older adolescents and young adults.[43]

CLINICAL FORMULATION
Predisposing Factors

BN is associated with numerous predisposing factors,[45] with research most consistently supporting genetic risk, gender (female), obstetric complications and perinatal factors, higher body mass index, experiences of sexual abuse or neglect during childhood, a cluster of factors around negative affect/psychiatric morbidity/neuroticism, diminished interoceptive awareness, escape-avoidance style of coping, and increased weight and shape concerns.

Precipitating Factors

The most commonly noted precipitating factors involve the developmental challenges inherent in entering puberty, and moving from adolescence to adulthood. Twin research indicates a significant increase in the expression of genetic risk appearing at puberty and early adulthood as well as new nonshared environmental factors at each time point.[46,47] The impact of these transitions is more difficult when accompanied by the experience of adverse life events or peer teasing about appearance,[48] where the former is also a potent trigger of genetic susceptibility to disordered eating.[49] These events are typically associated with feelings of low self-esteem, ineffectiveness, and difficulties with emotion regulation. Such experiences when layered on the internalization of the thin ideal and weight and shape concerns[50] can result in adhering to strict dietary rules to lose weight in order to accomplish important goals, including a desire to control life, feel effective, feel better about oneself, gain positive attention, and protect oneself emotionally. Dieting is a powerful immediate trigger of disordered eating.[51]

Perpetuating Factors

Often described as the "vicious cycle," the cognitive behavioral model of BN (**Fig. 1**) provides a depiction of perpetuating and maintaining factors that can be usefully shared with the patient. This general conceptualization provides a basis from which to develop a personalized cycle for the patient that can provide an individualized "road map" for effective treatment.

PROGNOSIS

In community samples, around 45% of patients can be expected to attain an asymptomatic status 14 years after initial onset,[12] with the remainder continuing to experience some symptoms; 14% will still be experiencing significant levels of disordered eating. The prior diagnosis of anorexia nervosa (regardless of age of

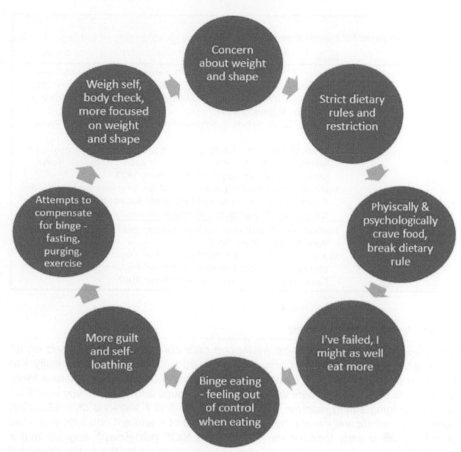

Fig. 1. The generic vicious cycle of BN.

onset or purging vs nonpurging subtype) decreases the likelihood of recovery from BN within 5 years.

TREATMENT
Meta-Analytic Results

Numerous treatment studies now exist for BN, as attested to by a body of meta-analytic studies. The most recent of these found that cognitive behavior therapy specific to eating disorders (CBT-ED) outperformed all other active psychological comparisons, including interpersonal psychotherapy.[52] A network meta-analysis that informed current NICE guidelines[39] concluded that the treatments most likely to achieve full remission are individual CBT-ED and guided self-help CBT-ED.[53] A comparison of CBT-ED and psychoanalytic psychotherapy unambiguously showed the former to be significantly more effective in decreasing binge eating and purging than the former, despite CBT-ED being of much shorter duration, N = 20 sessions over 5 months compared with weekly sessions over a 2-year period.[54] Resources for use in guided self-help and CBT-ED treatment manuals are summarized in **Table 3**.

Table 3 Treatment resources for bulimia nervosa	
Purpose	**Book**
Guided self-help	Cooper M, Todd G, Wells A. Bulimia nervosa: a cognitive therapy programme for clients. London: Jessica Kingsley Publishers; 2001.
	Cooper PJ. Bulimia nervosa and binge eating. A guide to recovery. London: Robinson; 1993.
	Fairburn CG. Overcoming binge eating. New York: Guilford Press; 1995.
	Schmidt U, Treasure J. Getting better bit(e) by bit(e). A survival kit for sufferers of bulimia nervosa and binge eating disorders. Hove: Lawrence Erlbaum Associates Publishers; 1993.
	Waller G, Mountford V, Lawson R, et al. Beating your eating disorder. A cognitive-behavioural self-help guide for adult sufferers and their carers. Cambridge: Cambridge University Press; 2010.
Individual CBT-ED, typically 20 sessions over 20 wk	Fairburn CG. Cognitive behaviour therapy and eating disorders. New York: Guilford Press; 2008.
	Waller G, Cordery H, Corstorphine E, et al. Cognitive behavioural therapy for eating disorders. A comprehensive treatment guide. Cambridge: Cambridge University Press; 2007.

Stepped Approach to Treatment

The NICE guidelines[39] emphasize a stepped care approach for BN, based on an accruing body of evidence. The provision of guided self-help CBT-ED, typically 4 to 9 sessions over 16 weeks, can be offered first. A robust finding across numerous treatment studies of eating disorders with different age groups is that if a therapy is ineffective for changing eating disorder behaviors over the first 4 sessions or weeks, then there will be significantly worse outcome at the end of treatment and follow-up than for the so-called early responders.[55] Hence the NICE guidelines[39] suggest that a change to a more intensive therapy should be considered by the fourth session if guided self-help CBT-ED is ineffective, contraindicated, or unacceptable. A demonstrative example of this was described by Chen and colleagues,[56] who entered women with binge-eating disorders (including BN) into guided self-help CBT-ED. Early strong responders (by session 4) continued in the guided self-help for up to 24 weeks (20- to 30-minute sessions), whereas the weak responders were randomized to either individualized CBT-ED or Dialectical Behavior Therapy, both involving 6 months of weekly sessions, a 2-hour group and 1-hour of individualized therapy. The weak responders "caught up" to the strong responders in terms of outcome by end of treatment and maintained this improvement at 6- and 12-month follow-up. The optimal intensity of a more intensive therapy option is unknown. Research suggests that, for some patients, a 10-session CBT-ED can be effective,[57] but to date, the type of patients this would suit is unknown. Further work on who does best with which treatment option is required in this area.

Promising Adjuncts

Although CBT-ED may be the current treatment of choice for BN, it is far from satisfactory in terms of outcome. A meta-analysis estimated that only 35% (95% confidence intervals: 29.6–41.7) of treatment completers achieved total symptom abstinence after receiving evidence-based treatments.[58] Current research is considering matching treatment adjuncts that may enhance outcomes for specific individuals, pointing to the need for an individualized approach to treatment selection. Although we are far from conclusions in this area, promising treatment adjuncts that need further investigation include imagery rescripting,[59] mindfulness,[60] dialectical skills training groups,[61] cognitive remediation training,[62] media literacy skills[63] training, and CBT for perfectionism.[64]

SUMMARY

Although there has been a decrease in the presentation of BN in primary care, there is an increase in disordered eating not meeting full diagnostic criteria that impacts adversely on long-term physical and psychological quality of life. Less than one-third of community cases of BN are detected by professionals due to a mix of patient ambivalence and shame, coupled with failure on the part of the professional to ask about or identify symptoms. Assessment should adopt a motivationally enhancing stance given the high level of ambivalence associated with BN, and the presence of self-harm and suicidality should be a routine component of assessment. CBT-ED out-performs other active psychological comparisons, but outcomes still require improvement. Future research should be directed at how to better match specific patients to various treatment approaches, especially with respect to suitable intensity and appropriate treatment adjuncts.

REFERENCES

1. American Psychiatric Association (APA). Diagnostic and statistical manual of mental disorders. 5th edition. Washington, DC: APA; 2013.
2. Fairburn CG, Cooper Z, O'Connor M. Eating disorder examination (16.0D). In: Fairburn CG, editor. Cognitive behavior therapy and eating disorders. New York: Guilford Press; 2008. p. 265–308.
3. American Psychiatric Association (APA). Diagnostic and statistical manual of mental disorders. 4th edition revised. Washington DC: APA; 2000.
4. Wade TD, Keski-Rahkonen A, Hudson J. Epidemiology of eating disorders. In: Tsuang M, Tohen M, editors. Textbook in psychiatric epidemiology. New York: Wiley; 2011. p. 343–60.
5. Smink FR, Van HD, Donker GA, et al. Three decades of eating disorders in Dutch primary care: decreasing incidence of bulimia nervosa but not anorexia nervosa. Psychol Med 2016;46:1189–96.
6. Keel PK, Heatherton TF, Dorer DJ, et al. Point prevalence of bulimia nervosa in 1982, 1992, and 2002. Psychol Med 2006;36:119–27.
7. Currin L, Schmidt U, Treasure J, et al. Time trends in eating disorder incidence. Br J Psychiatry 2005;186:132–5.
8. Hay PJ, Mond J, Buttner P, et al. Eating disorder behaviors are increasing: findings from two sequential community surveys in South Australia. PLos One 2008;3: e1541.
9. Wade TD, Wilksch SM, Lee C. A longitudinal investigation of the impact of disordered eating on young women's quality of life. Health Psychol 2012;31:352–9.
10. Favaro A, Caregaro L, Tenconi E, et al. Time trends in age of onset of anorexia nervosa and bulimia nervosa. J Clin Psychiatry 2009;70:1715–21.
11. Kessler RC, Berglund PA, Chiu WT, et al. The prevalence and correlates of binge eating disorder in the World Health Organization World Mental Health Surveys. Biol Psychiatry 2013;73:904–14.

12. Wade TD, Bergin JL, Tiggemann M, et al. Prevalence and long-term course of lifetime eating disorders in an adult Australian twin cohort. Aust N Z J Psychiatry 2006;40:121–8.
13. Keski-Rahkonen A, Hoek HW, Linna MS, et al. Incidence and outcomes of bulimia nervosa: a nationwide population-based study. Psychol Med 2009;39:823–31.
14. Keski-Rahkonen A, Mustelin L. Epidemiology of eating disorders in Europe: prevalence, incidence, comorbidity, course, consequences, and risk factors. Curr Opin Psychiatry 2016;29:340–5.
15. Preti A, Rocchi MB, Sisti D, et al. Comprehensive meta-analysis of the risk of suicide in eating disorders. Acta Psychiatr Scand 2011;12:6–17.
16. Franko D, Keel P. Suicidality in eating disorders: occurrence, correlates, and clinical implications. Clin Psychol Rev 2006;26:769–82.
17. Bulik CM, Sullivan PF, Joyce PR. Temperament, character and suicide attempts in anorexia nervosa, bulimia nervosa and major depression. Acta Psychiatr Scand 1999;100:27–32.
18. Forcano L, Fernandez-Aranda F, Alvarez-Moya E, et al. Suicide attempts in bulimia nervosa: personality and psychopathological correlates. Eur Psychiatry 2009;24:91–7.
19. Favaro A, Santonastaso P. Suicidality in eating disorders: clinical and psychological correlates. Acta Psychiatr Scand 1997;95:508–14.
20. Lavender JM, Wonderlich SA, Engel SG, et al. Dimensions of emotion dysregulation in anorexia nervosa and bulimia nervosa: a conceptual review of the empirical literature. Clin Psychol Rev 2015;40:111–22.
21. Lavender JM, Mitchell JE. Eating disorders and their relationship to impulsivity. Curr Treat Options Psychiatry 2015;2:394–401.
22. Fischer S, Smith GT, Cyders MA. Another look at Impulsivity: a meta-analytic review comparing specifics dispositions to rash action in their relationship to bulimic symptoms. Clin Psychol Rev 2008;28:1413–25.
23. Wade TD, Bulik CM, Prescott C, et al. Sex influences on shared risk factors for bulimia nervosa and other psychiatric disorders. Arch Gen Psychiatry 2004;61:251–6.
24. Baker JH, Mazzeo SE, Kendler KS. Association between broadly defined bulimia nervosa and drug use disorders: common genetic and environmental influences. Int J Eat Disord 2007;40:673–8.
25. Baker JH, Mitchell KS, Neale MC, et al. Eating disorder symptomatology and substance use disorders: prevalence and shared risk in a population based twin sample. Int J Eat Disord 2010;43:648–58.
26. Klabunde M, Collado D, Bohon C. An interoceptive model of bulimia nervosa: a neurobiological systematic review. J Psychiatr Res 2017;94:36–46.
27. Fairburn CG, Harrison P. Eating disorders. Lancet 2003;361:407–16.
28. Rodgers RF, Paxton SJ, McLean SA, et al. Stigmatizing attitudes and beliefs toward bulimia nervosa: the importance of knowledge and eating disorder symptoms. J Ner Ment Dis 2015;203:259–63.
29. Mond JM, Arrigi A. Perceived acceptability of anorexia and bulimia in women with and without eating disorder symptoms. Aust J Psychol 2012;64:108–17.
30. McLean SA, Paxton SJ, Massey R, et al. Stigmatizing attitudes and beliefs about bulimia nervosa: gender, age, education and income variability in a community sample. Int J Eat Disord 2014;47:353–61.
31. Fursland A, Watson HJ. Eating disorders: a hidden phenomenon in outpatient mental health? Int J Eat Disord 2014;47:422–5.

32. Currin L, Waller G, Treasure J, et al. The use of guidelines for dissemination of 'best practice' in primary care of patients with eating disorders. Int J Eat Disord 2007;40:476–9.

33. Pearson C, Smith GT. Bulimic symptom onset in young girls: a longitudinal trajectory analysis. J Abnorm Psychol 2015;24:1003–13.

34. Wilksch SM, Wade TD. Risk factors for clinically significant importance of shape and weight in adolescent girls. J Abnorm Psychol 2010;119:206–15.

35. Wade TD, Pellizzer M. Assessment of eating disorders. In: Sellbom M, Suhr J, editors. Cambridge handbook of clinical assessment and diagnosis. Cambridge (England): Cambridge University Press; 2018.

36. Rollnick S, Miller WR, Butler CC, editors. Motivational interviewing in health care: helping patients change behavior. New York: Guilford Press; 2008.

37. Miller WR, Rollnick S. Talking oneself into change: motivational interviewing, stages of change, and therapeutic process. J Cog Psychother 2004;18(4):299–308.

38. Steele AL, Bergin JL, Wade TD. Self-efficacy as a robust predictor of outcome in guided self-help treatment for broadly-defined Bulimia Nervosa. Int J Eat Disord 2011;44:389–96.

39. NICE. Eating disorders: recognition and treatment. (NC69). 2017. Available at: https://www.nice.org.uk/guidance/ng69. Accessed November 2, 2018.

40. Linardon J, Wade TD, de la Piedad GX, et al. Psychotherapy for bulimia nervosa on symptoms of depression: a meta-analysis of randomized controlled trials. Int J Eat Disord 2017;50:1124–36.

41. Mitchell JE, Crow S. Medical complications of anorexia nervosa and bulimia nervosa. Curr Opin Psychiatry 2006;19:438–43.

42. Mannucci E, Rotella F, Ricca V, et al. Eating disorders in patients with type 1 diabetes: a meta-analysis. J Endocrinol Invest 2005;28:417–9.

43. Rydall AC, Rodin GM, Olmsted MP, et al. Disordered eating behavior and microvascular complications in young women with insulin-dependent diabetes mellitus. N Eng J Med 1997;336:1849–54.

44. Polonsky WH, Anderson BJ, Lohrer PA, et al. Insulin omission in women with IDDM. Diabetes Care 1994;17:1178–85.

45. Jacobi C, Fittig E. Psychosocial risk factors for eating disorders. In: Agras S, editor. The oxford handbook of eating disorders. New York: Oxford University Press; 2010. p. 123–36.

46. Klump KL, Burt SA, McGue M, et al. Changes in genetic and environmental influences on disordered eating across adolescence: a longitudinal twin study. Arch Gen Psychiatry 2007;64:1409–15.

47. Fairweather-Schmidt AK, Wade TD. Changes in genetic and environmental influences on disordered eating between early and late adolescence: a longitudinal twin study. Psychol Med 2015;45:3249–58.

48. Wade TD, Hansell NK, Crosby RD, et al. A study of changes in genetic and environmental influences on weight and shape concern across adolescence. J Abnorm Psychol 2013;22:119–30.

49. Fairweather-Schmidt AK, Wade TD. Does peer-teasing moderate genetic and environmental risk for disordered eating? Br J Psychiatry 2017;201:350–5.

50. Fairweather-Schmidt AK, Wade TD. Characterizing and predicting trajectories of disordered eating over adolescence. J Abnorm Psychol 2016;125:369–80.

51. Stice E, Gau JM, Rohde P, et al. Risk factors that predict future onset of each DSM-5 eating disorder: predictive specificity in high-risk adolescent females. J Abnorm Psychol 2017;126:38–51.

52. Linardon J, Wade TD, de la Piedad GX, et al. The efficacy of cognitive-behavioral therapy for eating disorders: a systematic review and meta-analysis. J Consult Clin Psychol 2017;85:1080–94.
53. Slade E, Keeney E, Mavranezouli I, et al. Treatments for bulimia nervosa: a network meta-analysis. Psychol Med 2018;1–8.
54. Poulsen S, Lunn S, Daniel SI, et al. A randomized controlled trial of psychoanalytic psychotherapy or cognitive-behavioral therapy for bulimia nervosa. Am J Psychiatry 2014;171:109–16.
55. Vall E, Wade TD. Predictors of treatment outcome in individuals with eating disorders: a systematic review and meta-analysis. Int J Eat Disord 2015;48:946–71.
56. Chen EY, Cacioppo J, Fettich K, et al. An adaptive randomized trial of dialectical behaviour therapy and cognitive behaviour therapy for binge eating. Psychol Med 2017;47:703–17.
57. Waller G, Tatham M, Turner H, et al. A 10-session cognitive behavioral therapy (CBT-T) for eating disorders: outcomes from a case series of non-underweight adult patients. Int J Eat Disord 2018;51:262–9.
58. Linardon J, Wade TD. How many individuals achieve symptom abstinence following psychological treatments for bulimia nervosa? A meta-analytic review. Int J Eat Disord 2018;51:287–94.
59. Pennesi J-L, Wade TD. Imagery rescripting and cognitive dissonance: a randomized controlled trial of two brief online interventions for women at risk of developing an eating disorder. Int J Eat Disord 2018;51:439–48.
60. Atkinson MJ, Wade TD. Mindfulness training. In: Tylka TL, Piran N, editors. Handbook of positive body image: constructs, protective factors, and interventions. Oxford (England): Oxford University Press; 2018.
61. Hill DM, Craighead LW, Safer DL. Appetite-focused dialectical behavior therapy for the treatment of binge eating with purging: a preliminary trial. Int J Eat Disord 2011;44:249–61.
62. Tchanturia K. Remediation Therapy (CRT) for eating and weight disorders. New York: Routledge; 2014.
63. Wilksch SM, O'Shea A, Taylor CB, et al. Online prevention of disordered eating in at-risk young-adult women: a two-country pragmatic randomised controlled trial. Psychol Med 2018;48(12):2034–44.
64. Steele AL, Wade TD. A randomised trial investigating guided self-help to reduce perfectionism and its impact on bulimia nervosa. Behav Res Ther 2008;46:1316–23.

Binge-Eating Disorder

Anja Hilbert, PhD

KEYWORDS

• Eating disorder • Binge eating • Obesity • Diagnosis • Treatment

KEY POINTS

• Binge-eating disorder is a clinical eating disorder characterized by recurrent binge eating in the absence of regular compensatory behaviors to prevent weight gain.
• Being the most frequent eating disorder, binge-eating disorder cooccurs with significant psychopathology, mental and physical comorbidity, obesity, and life impairment.
• Despite its significance, binge-eating disorder is not sufficiently recognized, diagnosed, and treated.
• Evidence-based treatments for binge-eating disorder mainly include psychotherapy and structured self-help treatment, with cognitive-behavioral therapy being the most well-established approach, as well as pharmacotherapy.
• Lisdexamfetamine is Food and Drug Administration approved for binge-eating disorder with a limitation of use.

Binge-eating disorder (BED) was first included as its own diagnostic entity in the *Fifth Edition of the Diagnostic and Statistical Manual of Mental Disorders (DSM-5)* within the Feeding and Eating Disorders section.[1] BED's hallmark feature is recurrent binge eating, involving the consumption of an amount of food that is definitively larger than what others would eat under comparable circumstances within a certain time, associated with a feeling of loss of control over eating. Diagnosis of BED according to *DSM-5* (307.59) requires this objective binge eating to occur at least once per week over 3 months. In contrast to binge eating in bulimia nervosa, binge eating in BED occurs without regular inappropriate compensatory behaviors aimed at preventing weight gain, such as self-induced vomiting, fasting, or laxative misuse. Binge eating in BED is further characterized by behavioral abnormalities, such as eating rapidly or until feeling uncomfortably full, and results in marked distress.

Disclosure Statement: Dr A. Hilbert received honoraria as a consultant from Popewoodhead, Globaldata, and Weight Watchers and published books about cognitive-behavioral therapy with Hogrefe.
Funded by: German Federal Ministry of Education and Research grant number: 01EO1501.
Integrated Research and Treatment Center AdiposityDiseases, Department of Medical Psychology and Medical Sociology, Department of Psychosomatic Medicine and Psychotherapy, University of Leipzig Medical Center, Philipp-Rosenthal-Strasse 27, Leipzig 04103, Germany
E-mail address: anja.hilbert@medizin.uni-leipzig.de

The *DSM-5* offers 2 specifications for the diagnosis of BED: current severity as indicated by the weekly frequency of binge eating; and partial or full remission status after meeting full criteria of BED. In addition, within the Other Specified Feeding or Eating Disorders, *DSM-5* newly defines a lower-threshold form of BED (307.59), also associated with significant distress or impairment in life functioning: BED of low frequency and/or limited duration can be diagnosed if objective binge eating is occurring less than once per week and/or for shorter than 3 months, while all other *DSM-5* criteria of BED still need to be met.

The *International Classification of Diseases and Related Health Problems, Tenth Edition (ICD-10)*[2] subsumed BED under the Other Eating Disorders (F50.8), without any further specific diagnostic criteria. For the Eleventh Edition of *ICD (ICD-11)*, scheduled for 2019, BED was designated its own eating disorder diagnosis. Deviating from the *DSM-5*, the *ICD-11* diagnosis of BED was proposed to be broadened and based on both objective and subjective binge eating, termed "loss of control eating." Loss of control eating is characterized as eating an objectively or subjectively large amount of food, while experiencing a sense of loss of control over eating. Although the sense of loss of control is a well-validated feature of binge eating, it has been cautioned that the size of a binge provides only incremental information in the explanation of illness severity and psychopathology in diverse eating disorders,[3] so that the clinical significance of this proposed diagnosis of BED may be decreased.

CLINICAL PRESENTATION

Establishing BED as its own diagnostic entity in *DSM-5*[1] was based on extant literature demonstrating the clinical significance of this disorder. Individuals with BED suffer from increased eating disorder (eg, weight and shape concern) and general psychopathology (eg, depressiveness, anxiety), and high comorbidity with mood disorders, anxiety disorders, and substance use disorders, and personality disorders, notably borderline personality disorder, when compared with individuals without BED, and individuals with or without obesity. In addition, BED frequently cooccurs with attention-deficit/hyperactivity disorder.[4] Thus, BED displays similar psychological impairments as the other well-defined eating disorders, anorexia nervosa and bulimia nervosa.

In addition to psychological comorbidity, BED frequently cooccurs with obesity (body mass index, BMI $\geq$30.0 kg/m^2). Because of this comorbidity, individuals with BED have an increased risk of the obesity-related medical sequelae, for example, type 2 diabetes mellitus, hypertension, and dyslipidemia, and of premature mortality.[5,6] Further health conditions increased in individuals with BED include asthma, gastrointestinal symptoms, sleep and pain disorders, neurologic problems, and gynecologic conditions.[7,8]

The eating behavior in BED is characterized by a general tendency toward overeating. In laboratory test meal studies, individuals with BED overate during both binge-eating and non-binge-eating meals when compared with weight-matched controls.[9] They described more variable meal patterns, including more snacking, nibbling, or double meals.[10] When compared with bulimia nervosa, individuals with BED displayed lower dietary restraint and actual restriction,[11] although they exhibited a pronounced body image disturbance.[12] Furthermore, they indicated greater craving, emotional eating, eating for coping purposes,[13] and greater hedonic hunger than controls, and thus, experience a greater motivation to eat for pleasure while not in caloric need.[14]

BED results in significant decreases in health-related quality of life and social function impairment, which is similar to the other defined eating disorders.[15,16] Also underlining the severity of this disorder, BED is associated with increased health care utilization and related costs,[15] often years before being diagnosed with BED.[17]

EPIDEMIOLOGY

BED is the most prevalent eating disorder. A representative community-based investigation of 36,306 adults in the United States with a primary focus on alcohol use disorder documented prevalence estimates of lifetime BED according to the *DSM-5* of 0.9%, and 12-month estimates of 0.4%.[16] In a further representative community sample of 6041 Australian adolescents and adults, the point prevalence of BED (*DSM-5*) amounted to 5.6%.[18] In addition, BED of low frequency and/or limited duration had a prevalence rate of 6.9%. Other population-based prevalence estimates of BED tend to fall in between these rates.[19]

BED presents with a distinct sociodemographic profile, when compared with anorexia nervosa and bulimia nervosa, including a more balanced gender ratio, higher rates of obesity, later age of onset, and longer duration of eating disorder symptoms.[19] For example, Udo and Grilo[16] found a 2 to 3 times increased odds for women to be affected by BED than men, a more than 2-fold increased odds for obesity, a mean age of onset of 24.5 years, and a mean duration of eating disorder symptoms of 15.9 years. BED generally occurs among diverse ethnic and/or racial backgrounds.[20] Longitudinal developmental community studies suggest a peak onset of BED in early adolescence in addition to a peak onset in early adulthood.[21,22]

ETIOLOGY

BED develops along a complex etiology involving multiple psychological, biological, and sociocultural influences.[23] Retrospective correlates of risk for BED were mostly shared with the other eating disorders and included premorbid negative affectivity, perfectionism, conduct problems, substance abuse, childhood obesity, family weight concerns and eating problems, parenting problems and family conflict, parental psychopathology, and physical and sexual abuse.[24]

A few longitudinal studies on the onset of BED indicated that childhood loss of control eating predicts development of BED in adolescence.[25,26] Risk factors longitudinally predicting BED onset in young women were overeating, body dissatisfaction, dieting, negative affect, and mental health impairment.[27] The sociocultural background of an idealization of thinness likely fosters perceived pressure to be thin and internalization of the thin ideal, which have been found to predict the onset of BED in adolescent girls.[28]

Formal genetic studies suggest a heritability of BED of about 41% to 57%, independent of obesity.[29,30] Molecular genetics research focusing on genes related to reward processing, homeostatic control, and mood processing is limited. Candidate gene studies have indicated the involvement of both dopamine (eg, DRD2) and μ-opioid (eg, OPRM1) receptor genes in the etiology of BED. Thus, the risk for binge eating in BED may be conveyed through a hypersensitivity to reward, which is likely to foster binge eating given our current obesogenic environment with high availability of palatable, calorically dense processed foods. In contrast, research addressing an involvement of the melanocortin 4 receptor gene or of the serotonin transporter gene (5HTT) in BED has yielded inconsistent results.

Overall, in light of the complex etiology of BED, prospective studies testing mediational and interactional models may contribute to understanding how various risk factors work together.

MAINTENANCE

Emotional, social, and cognitive dysfunctions have been assumed to be maintaining factors of BED. According to the prominent affect regulation model,[31] binge-eating episodes are triggered by and serve to provide relief from negative affect. Indeed, descriptive, laboratory, and ecological momentary assessment studies confirmed binge eating in BED to be preceded by negative affect.[32] However, no clear evidence exists that binge eating actually reduces negative affect. Binge-eating episodes are likely to occur against a general background of a reduced emotional awareness and difficulties in emotion regulation, which were significantly more pronounced in BED versus weight-matched controls, and similar, albeit slightly less pronounced than in the other eating disorders.[33,34] Negative affect often arises from interpersonal problems that are reported more frequently by individuals with BED than controls.[35] Interpersonal problems were cross-sectionally found to be associated with eating disorder psychopathology, partially mediated by negative affect, thus lending some support to the interpersonal model of binge eating.[36]

Binge eating is further regarded as resulting from underlying neurocognitive dysfunctions, including difficulties in inhibitory control and reward processing, especially in the processing of disorder-relevant stimuli such as food cues, as determined using behavioral measures.[33,37–39] Neuroimaging studies, mostly based on functional magnetic resonance imaging, documented a related differential brain activation, for example, hypoactivity in prefrontal networks and hyperactivity in the medial orbitofrontal cortex when compared with weight-matched controls.[38,39] Current research on reward-based decision making showcased an impaired behavioral adaptation, including an increased switching behavior in BED when compared with weight-matched controls. This behavior was accompanied by reduced activation in the anterior insula/ventrolateral prefrontal cortex, typically associated with reversing behavior, and thus potentially relevant in the maintenance of binge eating despite its adverse consequences.[40] Negative mood seems to exacerbate inhibitory deficits in BED and resulted in less thorough conflict monitoring on the N2 component of electroencephalographic (EEG) event-related potentials and in more inhibition error deficits regarding food cues in an antisaccade task than in weight-matched and normal weight controls,[41] supporting an interaction of emotional and cognitive factors in the maintenance of BED.

Neurocognitive similarities of BED and obesity with substance use disorders resulted in the prominent, yet controversial food addiction hypothesis, according to which certain foods (eg, high sugar, high fat) may elicit addictive responses in vulnerable individuals with high impulsivity and reward sensitivity.[42] Although BED, viewed as an "eating addiction," and substance use disorders may share these vulnerabilities, other important characteristics are distinct: for example, substance use disorders are defined by specific addictive agent and symptoms of withdrawal or tolerance, none of which have been demonstrated regarding food.[11] Further critical aspects are that food addiction in humans is mainly operationalized through self-report and has unclear clinical relevance.

Overall, new research on the maintenance of BED should be used to refine clinical maintenance models providing treatment rationales, for example, the cognitive-behavioral model that was developed for bulimia nervosa,[43] without specifically adapting it to BED. Biopsychological aspects of the maintenance of binge eating await further clarification.

PROGNOSIS

Regarding long-term outcome, limited longitudinal evidence suggests that the natural course of BED is more variable than that in anorexia nervosa or bulimia nervosa, with tendencies toward recovery and relapse likely embedded in a chronic course.[44,45] Furthermore, BED seems to be less likely to migrate to another eating disorder diagnosis over time in community samples,[44,46] although in some clinical samples, an increased odds of migration to other eating disorder diagnoses, mostly bulimia nervosa, has been noted.

Little is known about the long-term mental or physical health outcome of BED. Significant negative mental health outcomes of binge-eating behaviors in youth are depressive symptoms and substance use.[26,47] Childhood binge-eating behaviors also predicted excess weight gain in adolescents,[47,48] as did diagnosis of BED in young women.[45] BED or binge-eating behaviors were found to independently increase the risk of the obesity-related sequelae in adolescents and adults, including metabolic symptoms.[7,8,48]

TREATMENT

A range of psychological and pharmacological treatments for patients with BED has been designed and evaluated in randomized-controlled trials (RCTs), with psychotherapy, self-help treatment, pharmacotherapy, behavioral weight loss (BWL) treatment, and combined treatment representing the most frequently evaluated treatment categories.

Psychotherapy

Current meta-analyses of RCTs in patients with BED demonstrated that psychotherapy, specifically the most frequently used approach of cognitive-behavioral therapy (CBT), has significant effects on the reduction of binge-eating episodes and remission from binge eating when compared with inactive control groups, mostly wait-list, at posttreatment.[49–51] In addition, psychotherapy significantly reduced eating disorder psychopathology, whereas effects on depression were inconsistent and weight loss effects were nonsignificant, indicating a stabilization of body weight. The long-term maintenance of effects was demonstrated in RCTs with CBT and interpersonal psychotherapy up to 4 years following treatment cessation.[52,53] A superiority of CBT over other conceptually and procedurally distinct psychotherapies that specifically addressed the symptoms of BED, for example, interpersonal psychotherapy or psychodynamic therapy, was not found.[50,54] Thus, although CBT is the most well-established psychotherapy for BED, other psychotherapies with specific interventions for BED may be as efficacious.

Structured Self-Help Treatment

Structured self-help treatment has mostly applied CBT manuals in book, electronic (eg, video), or Internet-based format, with or without guidance from a mental health professional. Meta-analyses of RCTs showed significant effects of self-help treatment on the reduction of binge-eating episodes and remission when compared with wait-list control conditions.[50,51] As with psychotherapy, eating disorder psychopathology was significantly improved when compared with wait-list control conditions. In contrast, effects on depression were inconsistent, and there were no significant effects on body weight. Long-term maintenance of effects in RCTs was found up to 24 months following treatment.[53,55] In comparative RCTs of guided versus unguided self-help treatment, differences in efficacy were not found.[50] Thus, guidance does not seem to be an indispensable element for patients with BED, although optimal intensity and types of guidance require further clarification. In comparative RCTs with psychotherapy, self-help treatment led to lower rates of remission from binge eating at follow-up and higher dropout, suggesting a lower efficacy and acceptance than in the more intense specialist psychotherapeutic treatment. In general, self-help treatment is a viable option helping many patients to fully remit from BED. It was found to be less costly than psychotherapy, however, not necessarily more cost-effective.[56] Further work is needed in this area.

Pharmacotherapy

For pharmacotherapy of BED, most RCTs used second-generation antidepressants (eg, fluoxetine), whereas a few RCTs used anticonvulsants (eg, topiramate) and the central nervous system stimulant lisdexamfetamine, the only medication approved by the Food and Drug Administration in 2015 for the treatment of BED.[49,50,57] Meta-analytically, pharmacotherapy using these agents outperformed pill placebo in most RCTs, showing significant effects on binge-eating episodes and remission. A significant weight loss effect was especially demonstrated for lisdexamfetamine,[49,50] whereas results on eating disorder psychopathology and depression were inconsistent. Data are lacking on long-term maintenance of effects and long-term administration. The incidence rate of adverse events and the related odds of premature discontinuation were significantly increased,[50] necessitating careful consideration in the pharmacotherapy of BED. Of note, lisdexamfetamine is marketed with a limitation of use, not being suited for weight loss and having a potential of serious cardiovascular adverse events.

Weight Loss Treatment

BWL treatment is not a treatment of BED, but represents the standard treatment of obesity, which is according to the 2013 Obesity Guideline generally indicated for individuals with BMI $\geq$30.0 kg/m^2 or for individuals with BMI $\geq$25 kg/m^2 (or increased waist circumference) and obesity-related comorbidities.[58] In a few RCTs, psychotherapy outperformed BWL treatment in reducing binge-eating episodes and eating disorder psychopathology at posttreatment and led to a significantly higher remission from binge eating at long-term follow-up.[50,59] Results were inconsistent as to whether BWL treatment produced a superior posttreatment weight loss outcome than psychotherapy, whereas at follow-up no differences were observed. Thus, BWL treatment was found to be less suited for the treatment of binge-eating symptomatology than psychotherapy. Other weight loss treatments that were evaluated in a few RCTs of BED are self-help weight loss treatment and antiobesity medications, such as orlistat.[50,57] Preliminary data suggest a decreased efficacy regarding binge-eating outcome in BED.

Combined Treatment

Combinations of CBT, BWL treatment, and/or pharmacological interventions did not show meta-analytical effects on binge-eating episodes and remission in RCTs, but eating disorder psychopathology, depression, and body weight were significantly reduced.[50] In direct comparisons, there were no differential effects of combined treatment versus psychotherapy on these outcomes, but a higher attrition from treatment was found. An additive effect being absent, combined treatment may be offered when psychotherapy alone is insufficient. However, combined treatment was superior to pharmacotherapy in reducing binge-eating episodes, but not in weight loss.[60] These results suggest that combined treatment may be favored over pharmacotherapy alone.

CONCLUSION

Psychotherapy, self-help treatment, and pharmacotherapy have empirical support in the treatment of BED. Because of the low quality of many RCTs for BED,[49,50] more high-quality research on diverse treatment approaches is warranted, with a focus on long-term maintenance and comparative efficacy. Pretreatment predictors informing about which patients with BED show a more favorable treatment response have not consistently been identified.[61] More research is also warranted on treatment-specific moderators, which could elucidate for whom a specific treatment works. The presumably most well-established treatment process factor for BED is rapid response.[62] Rapid response, typically defined as a 65% to 70% reduction in binge eating over the first 4 weeks of treatment, is a positive prognostic indicator of sustained remission from binge eating across a range of psychotherapeutic and self-help treatment approaches,[63] highlighting a particular relevance of monitoring a patient's response early in treatment.

FUTURE DIRECTIONS

Despite these clinical advances, BED is still not sufficiently being recognized, diagnosed, and treated.[64] For example, Kessler and colleagues[20] documented in 24,124 adults from 14 countries that only 38.3% of lifetime cases with BED ever received a specific treatment for their eating disorder. This "treatment gap" may be attributable to multiple system factors (eg, lack of screening for eating disorders) and patient factors (eg, lack of information, perceived stigma, shame).[65] Contributing to this gap, BED is publicly perceived as less impairing than the other eating disorders and attributable to a lack of self-discipline, which forms the basis of the stigma associated with BED.[66] Although it remains unclear how these stereotypes affect health care professionals' interventions for patients with BED, on the patients' side, perceived stigma is one major barrier to seek help for an eating disorder such as BED.[67] In addition, a "research-practice gap" was identified, including a discrepancy between evidence-based treatments and actual treatment delivery: For example, eating disorder therapists commonly offer eclectic combinations of interventions, not adhering to evidence-based treatment protocols.[68] These results highlight a substantial challenge of disseminating and implementing evidence-based treatments for BED into clinical practice.

In order to further increase the efficacy of evidence-based treatments for BED, current research on the nature or maintenance of this disorder warrants translation into new interventions and/or treatments. For example, interventions to improve inhibitory control, especially regarding disorder-relevant stimuli, may have potential, including technology-assisted bias modification training,[69] cue exposure,[70] or noninvasive neuromodulation using EEG neurofeedback.[71]

Regarding the classification of BED, further evidence is needed on its reliability and validity, taking into account the changes to diagnostic criteria in *DSM-5* and *ICD-11*. Difficulties exist in the differentiation of BED from other eating disorders, for example, bulimia nervosa with nonpurging compensatory behaviors. More research is warranted on the operationalization of diagnostic criteria, especially binge eating with its components of loss of control and size, the behavioral abnormalities, and severity rating. In addition, overvaluation of shape and weight, characteristic of the majority but not all individuals with BED, has been recommended, for example, as a diagnostic specifier, indicating greater illness severity.[72]

REFERENCES

1. American Psychiatric Association. Diagnostic and statistical manual of mental disorders. 5th edition. Arlington (VA): American Psychiatric Association; 2013.
2. World Health Organization. International classification of diseases and related health problems tenth edition (ICD-10). Geneva (Switzerland): World Health Organization; 1992.

3. Forney KJ, Bodell LP. Incremental validity of the episode size criterion in binge-eating definitions: an examination in women with purging syndromes. Int J Eat Disord 2016;49:651–62.
4. Ziobrowski H, Brewerton TD, Duncan AE. Associations between ADHD and eating disorders in relation to comorbid psychiatric disorders in a nationally representative sample. Psychiatry Res 2018;260:53–9.
5. Global BMI Mortality Cooperation, Di Angelantonio E, Bhupathiraju S, et al. Body-mass index and all-cause mortality: individual-participant-data meta-analysis of 239 prospective studies in four continents. Lancet 2016;388:776–86.
6. Ma C, Avenell A, Bolland M, et al. Effects of weight loss interventions for adults who are obese on mortality, cardiovascular disease, and cancer: systematic review and meta-analysis. BMJ 2017;359:j4849.
7. Mitchell JE. Medical comorbidity and medical complications associated with binge-eating disorder. Int J Eat Disord 2016;49:319–23.
8. Olguin P, Fuentes M, Gabler G, et al. Medical comorbidity of binge eating disorder. Eat Weight Disord 2017;22:13–26.
9. Heaner MK, Walsh BT. A history of the identification of the characteristic eating disturbances of bulimia nervosa, binge eating disorder and anorexia nervosa. Appetite 2013;71:445–8.
10. Masheb RM, Grilo CM, White MA. An examination of eating patterns in community women with bulimia nervosa and binge eating disorder. Int J Eat Disord 2011;44:618–24.
11. Schulte EM, Grilo CM, Gearhardt AN. Shared and unique mechanisms underlying binge eating disorder and addictive disorders. Clin Psychol Rev 2016;44:125–39.
12. Lewer M, Bauer A, Hartmann AS, et al. Different facets of body image disturbance in binge eating disorder: a review. Nutrients 2017;9:E1294.
13. Leslie M, Turton R, Burgess E, et al. Testing the addictive appetite model of binge eating: the importance of craving, coping, and reward enhancement. Eur Eat Disord Rev 2018;26:541–50.
14. Espel-Huynh HM, Muratore AF, Lowe MR. A narrative review of the construct of hedonic hunger and its measurement by the power of food scale. Obes Sci Pract 2018;4:238–49.
15. Agh T, Kovács G, Supina D, et al. A systematic review of the health-related quality of life and economic burdens of anorexia nervosa, bulimia nervosa, and binge eating disorder. Eat Weight Disord 2016;21:353–64.
16. Udo T, Grilo CM. Prevalence and correlates of DSM-5-defined eating disorders in a nationally representative sample of U.S. adults. Biol Psychiatry 2018;84:345–54.
17. Watson HJ, Jangmo A, Smith T, et al. A register-based case-control study of health care utilization and costs in binge-eating disorder. J Psychosom Res 2018;108:47–53.
18. Hay P, Girosi F, Mond J. Prevalence and sociodemographic correlates of DSM-5 eating disorders in the Australian population. J Eat Disord 2015;3:19.
19. Lindvall Dahlgren C, Wisting L, Rø Ø. Feeding and eating disorders in the DSM-5 era: a systematic review of prevalence rates in non-clinical male and female samples. J Eat Disord 2017;5:56.
20. Kessler RC, Berglund PA, Chiu WT, et al. The prevalence and correlates of binge eating disorder in the World Health Organization World Mental Health Surveys. Biol Psychiatry 2013;73:904–14.
21. Swanson SA, Crow SJ, Le Grange D, et al. Prevalence and correlates of eating disorders in adolescents. Results from the national comorbidity survey replication adolescent supplement. Arch Gen Psychiatry 2011;68:714–23.

22. Stice E, Marti CN, Rohde P. Prevalence, incidence, impairment, and course of the proposed DSM-5 eating disorder diagnoses in an 8-year prospective community study of young women. J Abnorm Psychol 2013;122:445–57.

23. Bakalar JL, Shank LM, Vannucci A, et al. Recent advances in developmental and risk factor research on eating disorders. Curr Psychiatry Rep 2015;17:42.

24. Hilbert A, Pike KM, Goldschmidt AB, et al. Risk factors across the eating disorders. Psychiatry Res 2014;220:500–6.

25. Hilbert A, Brauhardt A. Childhood loss of control eating over five-year follow-up. Int J Eat Disord 2014;47:758–61.

26. Tanofsky-Kraff M, Shomaker LB, Olsen C, et al. A prospective study of pediatric loss of control eating and psychological outcomes. J Abnorm Psychol 2011;120: 108–18.

27. Stice E, Gau JM, Rohde P, et al. Risk factors that predict future onset of each DSM-5 eating disorder: predictive specificity in high-risk adolescent females. J Abnorm Psychol 2017;126:38–51.

28. Stice E, Marti CN, Durant S. Risk factors for onset of eating disorders: evidence of multiple risk pathways from an 8-year prospective study. Behav Res Ther 2011; 49:622–7.

29. Mayhew AJ, Pigeyre M, Couturier J, et al. An evolutionary genetic perspective of eating disorders. Neuroendocrinology 2018;106:292–306.

30. Yilmaz Z, Hardaway JA, Bulik CM. Genetics and epigenetics of eating disorders. Adv Genomics Genet 2015;5:131–50.

31. Polivy J, Herman CP. Etiology of binge eating: psychological mechanisms. In: Fairburn CG, Wilson GT, editors. Binge eating: nature, assessment, and treatment. New York: Guilford Press; 1993. p. 173–205.

32. Nicholls W, Devonport TJ, Blake M. The association between emotions and eating behaviour in an obese population with binge eating disorder. Obes Rev 2016;17: 30–42.

33. Kittel R, Brauhardt A, Hilbert A. Cognitive and emotional functioning in binge-eating disorder: a systematic review. Int J Eat Disord 2015;48:535–54.

34. Dingemans A, Danner U, Parks M. Emotion regulation in binge eating disorder: a review. Nutrients 2017;9:E1274.

35. Brugnera A, Lo Coco G, Salerno L, et al. Patients with binge eating disorder and obesity have qualitatively different interpersonal characteristics: results from an Interpersonal Circumplex study. Compr Psychiatry 2018;85:36–41.

36. Ivanova IV, Tasca GA, Proulx G, et al. Does the interpersonal model apply across eating disorder diagnostic groups? A structural equation modeling approach. Compr Psychiatry 2015;63:80–7.

37. Giel KE, Teufel M, Junne F, et al. Food-related impulsivity in obesity and binge eating disorder-a systematic update of the evidence. Nutrients 2017;9:E1170.

38. Kessler RM, Hutson PH, Herman BK, et al. The neurobiological basis of binge-eating disorder. Neurosci Biobehav Rev 2016;63:223–38.

39. Kober H, Boswell RG. Potential psychological and neural mechanisms in binge eating disorder: implications for treatment. Clin Psychol Rev 2018;60:32–44.

40. Reiter AM, Heinze HJ, Schlagenhauf F, et al. Impaired flexible reward-based decision-making in binge eating disorder: evidence from computational modeling and functional neuroimaging. Neuropsychopharmacology 2017;42:628–37.

41. Leehr EJ, Schag K, Dresler T, et al. Food specific inhibitory control under negative mood in binge-eating disorder: evidence from a multimethod approach. Int J Eat Disord 2018;51:112–23.

42. Gearhardt AN, Davis C, Kuschner R, et al. The addiction potential of hyperpalatable foods. Curr Drug Abuse Rev 2011;4:140–5.
43. Fairburn CG, Cooper Z, Shafran R. Cognitive behaviour therapy for eating disorders: a "transdiagnostic" theory and treatment. Behav Res Ther 2003;41:509–28.
44. Agras WS, Crow S, Mitchell JE, et al. A 4-year prospective study of eating disorder NOS compared with full eating disorder syndromes. Int J Eat Disord 2009;42: 565–70.
45. Fairburn CG, Cooper Z, Doll HA, et al. The natural course of bulimia nervosa and binge eating disorder in young women. Arch Gen Psychiatry 2000;57:659–65.
46. Schaumberg K, Jangmo A, Thornton LM, et al. Patterns of diagnostic transition in eating disorders: a longitudinal population study in Sweden. Psychol Med 2018; 18:1–9.
47. Field AE, Sonneville KR, Micali N, et al. Prospective association of common eating disorders and adverse outcomes. Pediatrics 2013;130:e289–95.
48. Tanofsky-Kraff M, Yanovski SZ, Schvey NA, et al. A prospective study of loss of control eating for body weight gain in children at high risk for adult obesity. Int J Eat Disord 2009;42:26–30.
49. Brownley KA, Berkman ND, Peat CM, et al. Binge-eating disorder in adults: a systematic review and meta-analysis. Ann Intern Med 2016;165:409–20.
50. Hilbert A, Petroff D, Herpertz S, et al. Meta-analysis of the effectiveness of psychological and medical treatments for binge-eating disorder (MetaBED). J Consult Clin Psychol, in press.
51. Linardon J, Wade TD, de la Piedad Garcia X, et al. The efficacy of cognitive-behavioral therapy for eating disorders: a systematic review and meta-analysis. J Consult Clin Psychol 2017;85:1080–94.
52. Hilbert A, Bishop ME, Stein RI, et al. Long-term efficacy of psychological treatments for binge eating disorder. Br J Psychiatry 2012;200:232–7.
53. Wilson GT, Wilfley TE, Agras WS, et al. Psychological treatments of binge eating disorder. Arch Gen Psychiatry 2010;67:94–101.
54. Spielmans GI, Benish SG, Marin C, et al. Specificity of psychological treatments for bulimia nervosa and binge eating disorder? A meta-analysis of direct comparisons. Clin Psychol Rev 2013;33:460–9.
55. de Zwaan M, Herpertz S, Zipfel S, et al. Effect of internet-based guided self-help vs individual face-to-face treatment on full or subsyndromal binge eating disorder in overweight or obese patients. JAMA Psychiatry 2017;74:987–95.
56. König HH, Bleibler F, Friederich HC, et al. Economic evaluation of cognitive behavioral therapy and Internet-based guided self-help for binge-eating disorder. Int J Eat Disord 2018;51:155–64.
57. McElroy SL. Pharmacologic treatments for binge-eating disorder. J Clin Psychiatry 2017;1:14–9.
58. Jensen MD, Ryan DH, Apovian CM, et al. 2013 AHA/ACC/TOS guideline for the management of overweight and obesity in adults. J Am Coll Cardiol 2013;63: 2985–3023.
59. Palavras MA, Hay P, Filho CA, et al. The efficacy of psychological therapies in reducing weight and binge eating in people with bulimia nervosa and binge eating disorder who are overweight or obese. Nutrients 2017;9:E299.
60. Grilo CM, Reas DL, Mitchell JE. Combining pharmacological and psychological treatments for binge eating disorder: current status, limitations, and future directions. Curr Psychiatry Rep 2017;18:55.

61. Linardon J, de la Piedad Garcia X, Brennan L. Predictors, moderators, and me-diators of treatment outcome following manualised cognitive-behavioural therapy for eating disorders: a systematic review. Eur Eat Disord Rev 2017;25:3–12.

62. Brauhardt A, de Zwaan M, Hilbert A. The therapeutic process in psychological treatments for eating disorders: a systematic review. Int J Eat Disord 2014;47: 565–84.

63. Grilo CM. Psychological and behavioral treatments for binge-eating disorder. J Clin Psychiatry 2017;1:20–4.

64. Kornstein SG. Epidemiology and recognition of binge-eating disorder in psychi-atry and primary care. J Clin Psychiatry 2017;1:3–8.

65. Kazdin AE, Fitzsimmons-Craft EE, Wilfley DE. Addressing critical gaps in the treatment of eating disorders. Int J Eat Disord 2017;50:170–89.

66. Puhl R, Suh Y. Stigma and eating and weight disorders. Curr Psychiatry Rep 2015;17:552.

67. Ali K, Farrer L, Fassnacht DB, et al. Perceived barriers and facilitators towards help-seeking for eating disorders: a systematic review. Int J Eat Disord 2017; 50:9–21.

68. Waller G. Treatment protocols for eating disorders: clinicians' attitudes, concerns, adherence and difficulties delivering evidence-based psychological interven-tions. Curr Psychiatry Rep 2016;18:1–8.

69. Schmitz F, Svaldi J. Effects of bias modification training in binge eating disorder. Behav Ther 2017;48:707–17.

70. Ferrer-Garcia M, Gutierrez-Maldonado J, Pla-Sanjuanelo J, et al. A randomised controlled comparison of second-level treatment approaches for treatment-resistant adults with bulimia nervosa and binge eating disorder: assessing the benefits of virtual reality cue exposure therapy. Eur Eat Disord Rev 2017;25: 479–90.

71. Abnormalities in the EEG power spectrum in bulimia nervosa, binge-eating disor-der, and obesity: A systematic review. Blume M, Schmidt R, Hilbert A. Eur Eat Dis-ord Rev 2018. [Epub ahead of print].

72. Grilo CM. Why no cognitive body image feature such as overvaluation of shape/weight in the binge eating disorder diagnosis? Int J Eat Disord 2013;46:208–11.

Avoidant Restrictive Food Intake Disorder

Debra K. Katzman, MD, FRCPC[a],*, Mark L. Norris, MD, FRCPC[b], Nancy Zucker, PhD[c]

KEYWORDS

- Avoidant restrictive food intake disorder (ARFID)
- *Diagnostic and Statistical Manual of Mental* Disorders [fifth edition] *(DSM-5)*
- Feeding and eating disorders • Food avoidance • Food restriction

KEY POINTS

- Avoidant restrictive food intake disorder (ARFID) is a newly classified disorder in the "Feeding and Eating Disorders" section of the *Diagnostic and Statistical Manual of Mental Disorders* (fifth edition).
- The prevalence of ARFID among children and adolescents ranges from 1.5% to 23% among eating disorder day treatment and inpatient treatment settings.
- Children and adolescents with ARFID are younger, include a greater proportion of boys (although still predominantly girls), and have a longer duration of illness compared with patients with anorexia nervosa (AN).
- Patients with ARFID compared with those with AN have a greater likelihood of comorbid medical and/or psychiatric illness.
- Currently, there are no empirically validated treatments for ARFID.

DIAGNOSTIC CRITERIA AND CONTEXT

Avoidant restrictive food intake disorder (ARFID) is a newly classified disorder in the "Feeding and Eating Disorders" section of the *Diagnostic and Statistical Manual of Mental Disorders* (fifth edition) (*DSM-5*).[1] ARFID is a feeding or eating disturbance

The authors do not have any relationships with commercial or financial company that has a direct financial interest in subject matter or materials discussed in this article or with a company making a competing product. D.K. Katzman has research funding from National Institutes of Health (NIH) and funding from Wolters Kluwer as Senior Associate Editor of *Adolescent and Young Adult Health Care*. N. Zucker has research funding from NIH.
[a] Division of Adolescent Medicine, Department of Pediatrics, The Hospital for Sick Children and University of Toronto, 555 University Avenue, Toronto, Ontario M5G 1X8, Canada; [b] Division of Adolescent Medicine, Department of Pediatrics, The Children's Hospital of Eastern Ontario (CHEO), University of Ottawa, CHEO Research Institute, 401 Smyth Road, Ottawa, Ontario K1H 8L1, Canada; [c] Department of Psychiatry and Behavioral Sciences, Duke School of Medicine, Duke University, Duke Center for Eating Disorders, PO Box 3454, Durham, NC 27710, USA
* Corresponding author.
E-mail address: debra.katzman@sickkids.ca

Psychiatr Clin N Am 42 (2019) 45–57
https://doi.org/10.1016/j.psc.2018.10.003
0193-953X/19/© 2018 Elsevier Inc. All rights reserved.

psych.theclinics.com

that includes a heterogeneous clinical presentation that can result in significant weight loss, nutritional deficiency, dependence on enteral feeding or nutritional supplements, and/or marked interference in psychosocial functioning. Individuals with ARFID can only be diagnosed in the absence of weight or shape concerns. Furthermore, the feeding or eating disturbance cannot be explained by lack of available food or by an associated culturally sanctioned practice. The eating disturbance cannot occur exclusively during the course of anorexia nervosa (AN) or bulimia nervosa (BN), nor can it be attributable to a concurrent medical condition or be better explained by another mental disorder. If the eating disturbance occurs in the context of another condition or disorder, the severity of the eating disturbance must exceed that routinely associated with the condition or disorder and requires additional clinical attention.

The emergence of ARFID as a diagnostic category in the *DSM-5* resulted from several gaps recognized in the *DSM-IV* diagnostic category Feeding or Eating Disorders of Infancy and Early Childhood (FEDIC).[2] Among the most significant gap was the fact that patients with FEDIC could only be diagnosed in children up until the age of 6 years. Evolving research suggested the presence of an older cohort of individuals that lacked body image concerns but exhibited significant feeding disturbances. An additional concern was that the impairment resulting from significant food avoidance and/or restriction may be broader than encapsulated in the FEDIC diagnosis. FEDIC only captured eating or feeding issues that resulted in weight loss and/or growth impairment.[3] In some cases, other documented nutritional and psychosocial consequences caused impairment secondary to inadequate or poor nutrition.[3] For example, research on food selectivity revealed that often entire food groups were avoided (eg, protein) without influence on growth trajectory. Likewise, the child's limited food variety may be such that it severely limits the family's mobility, adds to family conflict, and/ or increases strain on the family system.[4,5] These impairing consequences were not captured with FEDIC. Finally, the diagnosis of FEDIC was rarely used and studied, and as such, there was limited information on the characteristics, course, and outcome of these children.

As a result, the FEDIC diagnosis was replaced with ARFID in the *DSM-5* as a means of capturing patients across the lifespan who have avoidant or restrictive eating that leads to significant medical or psychosocial problems and lack the body image concerns seen in individuals with AN and BN.[1]

EPIDEMIOLOGY

Currently, there is a paucity of epidemiologic data on patients with ARFID over the lifespan.

Before the establishment of ARFID as a diagnosis, 3 separate prospective pediatric surveillance studies were conducted to determine the incidence and age-specific presentation of early-onset restrictive eating disorders (EDs) in children in Australia, Canada, and the United Kingdom. A latent class analysis of the total sample revealed 2 distinct clinical clusters, both of which presented with food avoidance. Cluster 1 included 56% of the cases who presented with symptoms of weight preoccupation, fear of being fat, body image distortion, and overexercising. Cluster 2 included 25% of the cases and was more likely to present with a comorbid psychiatric disorder. Clusters 1 and 2 closely resembled the *DSM-5* criteria for AN and ARFID, respectively.[6]

After the diagnostic category of ARFID was established, the prevalence of this disorder in North American pediatric tertiary care ED programs was noted to be 5% to 14%. In contrast, the prevalence of ARFID in a pediatric ED day treatment program was reported to be 23%. One study looking at ARFID in a pediatric gastroenterology clinic found a prevalence rate of 1.5% of children and adolescents between 8 and 18 years. One or more ARFID symptoms were present in another 2.4% but a diagnosis could not definitely be made.[7] One community-based sample, using a self-report screening tool in 8 to 13 year olds, demonstrated features of ARFID in 3.2% of the study population.[8]

Most studies in patients with ARFID have been in pediatric samples. The inclusion of adults among those who can be diagnosed with ARFID has necessitated a new approach in conceptualizing this disorder. This new conceptualization of ARFID may in part explain why there are so few studies on the epidemiology of ARFID in adults. There are, however, a few case reports[9–11] that have described the disorder in adolescents and adults. A retrospective chart review in a Japanese sample of women with feeding and EDs ages 14 to 50[12] years identified 11% of patients who met the DSM-5 criteria for ARFID. The ARFID group had significantly shorter duration of illness, lower rates of admission history, and less severe psychopathology when compared with patients with AN. Finally, a community-based survey of individuals 15 years and older in South Australia found the 3-month prevalence of ARFID to be 0.3%.[13]

CLINICAL MANIFESTATIONS OF AVOIDANT RESTRICTIVE FOOD INTAKE DISORDER

A picture of the phenomenology of ARFID is emerging. Central to this understanding is the recognition that ARFID, being broad in its scope, captures various manifestations of food avoidance/restriction that may be distinct in pathophysiology and thus may necessitate diverse treatment approaches. The DSM-5 suggests motivations that may contribute to food avoidance/restriction: avoidance of foods due to their sensory properties (ie, taste, texture, smell), low appetite or disinterest in food, or fear of negative consequences from eating (ie, fear of choking or vomiting).[1] As with any example provided in a diagnostic document, there is a danger that these examples become reified and exclusive, thus other motivations for food avoidance become neglected. Notwithstanding, Norris and colleagues[12] reported that among a sample of 75 individuals who met criteria for ARFID, 3 subgroups could be identified corresponding to these distinct motivations for food avoidance, each with distinct associated features: (1) those with limited intake that were associated with lack of interest in eating/poor appetite; (2) those with limited variety associated with the sensory features of eating; and (3) those whose avoidance of eating had occurred in response to a specific event. Findings revealed that those with the limited variety/sensory aversion subtype had the longest length of illness (18% of the sample), whereas those who had experienced an aversive event (43%) were more likely to be admitted to a tertiary care center. Approximately 22% of this sample had a mixed presentation. Similar groups were reported when a developed measurement tool for ARFID was subject to factor analysis and included those with insufficient food quantity; those with insufficient variety; and those with avoidance after a traumatic event.[14] In a proposed model of the neurobiology of ARFID, Thomas and colleagues[15] suggest that although these motivations may have a distinct pathophysiology, the degree of these motivations may co-occur within an individual and thus may necessitate a blending of distinct approaches.

In addition, there also seems to be some common elements when examining cases of ARFID, particularly as the disorder becomes more severe. For example, Cooney and colleagues[16] completed a retrospective chart review of 31 individuals with ARFID presenting to a tertiary care center. Of these, 96.4% had experienced weight loss or failure to make expected gains, and 3.6% were dependent on nutritional supplements. All of these individuals had 2 or more physical symptoms with more than 50%

reporting abdominal pain. A history of nausea and early satiety were also present in most of the sample. Of interest, 71.4% described a triggering event for the avoidance despite a pattern of food avoidance that had been of long duration. Thus, for some, the diagnosis of ARFID may represent a worsening of food avoidance that crosses a threshold of impairment against a backdrop in which adequate intake or intake of optimal quality had been substandard for a long duration. Notably, most of the children had seen another specialist before presenting to a specialized ED program, suggesting challenges in the early recognition of ARFID.

An alternative strategy to understanding the clinical presentation of individuals with ARFID has been to compare cases of ARFID to cases of AN or BN. In general, populations of children and adolescents with ARFID compared with those with AN or BN were found to have a greater proportion of boys (although still predominantly girls) were younger and had a longer duration of illness. Furthermore, patients with ARFID were found to have a greater likelihood of comorbid medical and/or psychiatric illness compared with patients with AN.[17–19] Patients with ARFID have higher rates of obsessive compulsive disorder,[18,19] generalized anxiety,[7,18–20] autism spectrum disorder,[18] attention-deficit/hyperactivity disorder,[18,21] learning disorders,[18] and cognitive impairment.[18]

EVALUATION OF PATIENTS WITH AVOIDANT RESTRICTIVE FOOD INTAKE DISORDER
History

The goal of the initial history is to develop rapport between the patient and clinician, to establish a diagnosis, and to determine an appropriate treatment setting. Pediatric assessments usually entail direct interviews with the child and parents, both together and separately. A full comprehensive history usually requires gathering data from the patient's parents/caregivers, partner, and/or referring clinician.

Parental or family concerns regarding feeding issues and eating behaviors with or without weight loss should be assessed carefully by clinicians regardless of the age of the patient. Evolving evidence suggests that children and adolescents with ARFID have contact with multiple pediatric providers before a formal ED assessment takes place and are less likely to self-refer to an ED program as compared with those with AN or BN.[7,19,20] As such, patients with ARFID often present with complex and long-standing histories that include psychiatric, medical, psychological, and sociocultural influences. Consequently, a multidisciplinary team is often essential to establishing a diagnosis and addressing treatment needs. The multidisciplinary team can include, but is not limited to, physicians, mental health professionals, dietitians, speech language pathologists, and occupational therapists. Ultimately, the structure of the multidisciplinary team will depend on the geographic location and availability of skilled health care professionals.

To make a diagnosis of ARFID, a thorough developmental, feeding, nutritional, and psychosocial history is critical to fully understand how a patient's presentation impacts their current physical and psychological well-being. The clinician will first want to get a good understanding of why the patient and family have engaged the health care system at this particular time. The clinician should attempt to determine when the feeding issues were first identified as a concern and clarify the range, variety, type, and sensory characteristics (tastes, textures, smells) of acceptable foods. The patient's appetite signaling and indifference to food intake should also be explored. Furthermore, the clinician should determine the extent to which developmental (ie, early feeding experiences), intrinsic (ie, the presence of anxiety), as well as extrinsic (ie, a traumatic feeding–related event such a choking) factors contribute to energy intake and therefore affect physical and sexual growth and development. It is not un-common for caregivers to report high levels of distress and impairment as a result of feeding-related experiences. It is important to understand how this influences the feeding experience. For example, bullying, severe or repeated self-limiting illnesses, or feeding-specific traumatic events (ie, vomiting or choking) can result in restrictive nutritional intake. The clinician will want to understand how the patient has tolerated and progressed both physically and psychologically with respect to adding foods at varying developmental stages. In addition, it is important to explore how the individual's sociocultural factors and ethnic values may influence the expression of their eating behaviors. The risk and/or presence of nutritional deficiency can be screened for using an assessment of dietary intake. A 24-hour dietary recall by the individual and/or family member should include types of foods and beverages, portion sizes, specific foods or food groups, foods intentionally avoided, dietary calcium intake, and other complementary or alternative medicines or supplements. The diverse presentation of ARFID can lead to specific micronutrient malnutrition or protein-energy malnutrition. Furthermore, the clinician should inquire about whether the patient depends on enteral feeding or nutritional supplements to sustain adequate intake. Finally, the clinician must also determine the extent to which the eating disturbance causes marked interference with psychosocial functioning, such as eating with others, attending school or age-appropriate social situations, or sustaining relationships.

It is important to keep in mind that the motivation that drives the feeding disturbances in patients with ARFID must not be related to cognitive concerns regarding the effects of food on shape, weight, or size. In fact, patients with ARFID may report being upset or distressed by being too thin and want to gain weight.

For girls, a complete menstrual history is important to assess for primary or secondary amenorrhea, which can be a result of weight loss or a chronic health condition. A thorough and careful review of systems is essential to determine a differential diagnosis, to help identify potential or underlying comorbid medical and psychiatric disorders, and to recognize medical complications resulting from a diagnosis of ARFID.

Finally, it is important to ask about family medical and mental illness. Parents may provide history suggestive of similar feeding challenges in other family members. This information will not only lend weight to the patient's diagnosis but will also provide information about the patient's background.

Physical Examination

In addition to the history, a complete physical examination should be performed at the initial assessment. The physical examination should include measurements of the patient's height and weight, and determination of body mass index (BMI = weight [kg]/height [m^2]). Previous heights and weights are also helpful. Weights and heights should be plotted on an age-appropriate growth curve for children and adolescents. This information is necessary to help determine the patient's treatment goal weight (TGW) and to detect compromised growth and development.[22,23] In addition, orthostatic heart rate and blood pressure should be checked as well as an oral temperature. A full and detailed physical examination, including sexual maturity rating, is necessary to help rule out medical causes of weight loss and/or growth impairment. Finally, the clinician should look for clinical findings consistent with nutritional deficiencies.

Laboratory Investigations

Laboratory assessment, including markers of nutritional deficiency, is an important component of a comprehensive workup. Laboratory assessments to consider in patients suspected of having a diagnosis of ARFID include complete blood count with differential, serum electrolytes, blood urea nitrogen and creatinine, liver function tests, thyroid-stimulating hormone, electrocardiogram (ECG), and dual x-ray absorptiometry. For girls who present with amenorrhea, a pregnancy test (human chorionic gonadotropin) should be performed. A history that suggests inadequate nutritional intake may prompt the need for further diagnostic workup[24–27]; in such cases, dietary deficiencies (ie, iron, calcium, vitamin B12, vitamin D, folate) should be explored. Depending on the history, erythrocyte sedimentation rate or C-reactive protein may help detect inflammation. Further diagnostic evaluation, such as a more extensive laboratory assessment, brain imaging, or procedural investigations (ie, endoscopy, barium swallow), may be indicated to exclude other suspected medical or psychiatric diagnoses that could present with signs and symptoms of ARFID.

PSYCHOLOGICAL INSTRUMENTS

The epidemiology, psychopathology, course, and outcome of patients with ARFID are limited by the lack of validated instruments. Diagnostic instruments are currently under development. A recent retrospective chart review on patients less than 18 years of age who were clinically diagnosed with ARFID found that commonly used pediatric ED psychometric measures lacked sensitivity in making a diagnosis of ARFID.[16] The results from this study however, do not refute the inclusion of ED-specific measures during a pediatric ED assessment because they can be helpful in the diagnosis of children and adolescents with AN.

The Eating Disturbances in Youth-Questionnaire is a 14-item, self-report measure originally developed to screen for early-onset restrictive eating disturbances in nonclinical populations. A Swiss population-based study of 8 to 13 year olds demonstrated good psychometric properties, including adequate discriminant and convergent validity of this tool.[8] A more recent principal component analysis (Zickgraf HF, 2018, personal communication) revealed a 4-factor structure, covering the 3 different restrictive eating disturbances and weight problems proposed in the *DSM-5* ARFID diagnostic category.[14]

The Pica, ARFID, Rumination Disorder Interview (PARDI) is a structured, multi-informant interview (parent version for 2–3 year olds; parent version for children aged 4 and over; self version for 8–13 year olds; and self version for those aged 14 years and older) that is being evaluated for the diagnosis of ARFID.[28] The PARDI provides details on the overall severity of ARFID and assessment of the 3 motivations outlined in *DSM-5*.

More recently, the 9-item ARFID screen (NIAS), a brief multidimensional instrument to measure ARFID-associated eating behaviors, was validated (for individuals 18 years and older) for 4 structures (picky eating, appetite, fear of negative consequences, and psychopathology) using exploratory and confirmatory factor analyses.[29] Currently, a parent-report version of the NIAS for children 5 to 17 years old is being tested (Zickgraf HF, 2018, personal communication).

Ultimately, a clinical interview with the patient and family by a mental health professional is the tool that will help make an accurate diagnosis of ARFID.

MEDICAL COMPLICATIONS

Patients with ARFID are at risk of medical complications secondary to malnutrition. Previous studies have demonstrated that outpatients with ARFID exhibit similar rates of weight loss and malnutrition as patients with AN.[18–20,30] Given the preponderance of low-weight patients with ARFID, it stands to reason that this group would also be at risk for the acute and chronic effects of malnutrition. There is evidence that patients with ARFID are susceptible to develop bradycardia, prolonged QT interval on ECG, and electrolyte abnormalities.[31] In fact, patients with ARFID have presented with rates of electrolyte abnormalities that are more than doubled those observed in AN.[31] In addition, patients with ARFID are at risk of menstrual irregularities[30] and amenorrhea.[32] Although there are no prospective studies examining the impact of ARFID on bone mineral density (BMD), one retrospective study demonstrated that 77% of patients with ARFID had BMD scores at least one standard deviation from the mean, with 25% reported to be in the osteoporotic range. BMD was significantly lower in the ARFID group compared with patients with AN (Norris, 2014).[20] Most studies in children and adolescents with EDs have shown that the ARFID cohort is younger than the non-ARFID cohort. As such, the reported malnutrition described in the patients with ARFID has the potential to impact physical and sexual growth and development.[18,19]

Studies have shown that patients with ARFID are less likely to be hospitalized than those with AN due to medical instability.[18–20,30] However, a recent study that looked at the utility of ARFID subtype assignments demonstrated that patients with traumatic feeding-related experiences were admitted into tertiary care centers more frequently than patients with primary sensory difficulties or low appetite/indifference to eating.[12] This observation suggests potential differences in the degree of medical morbidity among ARFID subtypes at first presentation.

TREATMENT

To date, there is a lack of empirically validated treatments for patients with ARFID across each level of care. Because the treatment needs of patients with ARFID are diverse, the multidisciplinary team should approach treatment in a way that best meets the patient's medical, nutritional, mental health, and feeding-specific needs while at the same time mitigating distress and impairment. Similar to the treatment approach in patients with AN, patients with ARFID that are malnourished, underweight, and/or growth impaired should be placed on adequate nutrition to reestablish weight restoration to the patient's TGW as quickly as possible.[22,23] Given the anxiety, food restrictions, and aversions present in many patients with ARFID, a thoughtful and compassionate approach to treatment is critical.

A current consideration is whether patients with ARFID require a unique and specialized therapeutic milieu and treatment program separate from other ED patients. For example, patients with ARFID and AN may have different nutritional requirements with respect to diet quality and quantity, which may make it challenging to have the same milieu structure apply to both groups. In addition, individuals with ARFID may view the "safe" foods of those with AN as "disgusting," whereas patients with AN may find the food and eating behaviors of those with ARFID "triggering." The risk is that these differences make the treatment milieu feel unsafe for patients, which is an important consideration. Furthermore, patients with ARFID may feel misunderstood by groups that emphasize body image. On the other hand, having different types of EDs treated in the same specialized day treatment program or inpatient unit assures a skilled ED staff, a safe and supportive environment that is sensitive to the needs of patients with EDs and may be more financially efficient. These issues need further study.

Medical Inpatient Treatment

Currently, many clinicians use the criteria for medical instability delineated for patients with restrictive EDs for their patients with ARFID.[22] Patients found to be medically unstable will require hospitalization. In such cases, a refeeding protocol is recommended. Peebles and colleagues[33] described an aggressive pediatric inpatient renourishment program that resulted in similar rates of weight gain and need for referral to higher levels of care in patients with ARFID and AN. Of note, individuals with ARFID were more likely to require use of nasogastric tube (NGT) feedings to restore nutrition and at younger ages relative to other ED diagnoses. The protocol included a meal plan with embedded "exposures" to increase the approach to feared foods in AN. However, the more frequent use of NGT feedings in children with ARFID suggested that the typical hospital meal plan was viewed as more challenging in this group.

The more frequent use of NGT feedings in ARFID raises some clinical concerns. Although NGT feedings may at times be a medical necessity, there is a potential danger that this treatment could be iatrogenic in that the aversive oral sensations of tube feedings in individuals who are already sensitive to oral sensations may lead to further conditioned food avoidance. Thus, although some ED programs may use this strategy as a routine technique when an individual fails to consume all or part of their prescribed meal, its use should be used more cautiously in individuals with ARFID.

Day Hospital Treatment

Day hospital or partial hospital programs provide an intermediate level of care between inpatient and outpatient treatment. One study compared the outcomes of patients with ARFID to those with other EDs in a day treatment setting.[21] They found that patients with ARFID had higher rates of NGT feedings and spent significantly fewer weeks in a program than those with AN. However, patients with ARFID experienced similar increases in % mean BMI as patients with AN and other specified/unspecified feeding and EDs. All patients exhibited significant improvements in eating attitudes and behaviors over the course of treatment, suggesting that patients with ARFID can be successfully treated among children with other EDs in the same day hospital setting.

Outpatient Psychological Treatment

There have been several single-case studies, nonrandomized group trials, and a limited number of randomized controlled trials investigating the efficacy of behavioral management approaches to increase food consumption in childhood feeding and EDs.[34,35] In general, thoughtful behavioral approaches can improve acute intake or eating behaviors across a variety of feeding and ED presentations as evidenced in rigorous single-case designs.[36] In one review, most interventions used escape extinction (ie, not removing the spoon until a bite is taken) with differential reinforcement of a behavior that is desired to be increased. Many of these strategies were examined in children with developmental disabilities or neurodevelopmental disorders. Although basic behavioral learning principles apply to everyone, what is rewarding, relieving, or punishing varies greatly across individuals based on nuanced considerations, including developmental capacities for learning. Furthermore, addressing caregiver burden and acceptability is crucial. Sharp and colleagues[37] used a multidisciplinary intervention that included graduated weaning of supplement feeds, escape extinction, reinforcement procedures, and a formalized meal structure over a 5-day interval among 1 to 6 year olds with ARFID. Acceptability and feasibility ratings by parents were extremely high, and the amount of food consumption was significantly improved relative to a waitlist control group. Other notable outpatient treatment examples include a pilot study that used appetite manipulation via medication, tube weaning, and pain management resulting in 100% of individuals weaned from tube feeding in a 14-week intervention.[38] This intervention may have decreased the aversive experiences of eating via pain management while increasing the rewarding value of food by increasing appetite. Knowledge of the relative effectiveness of these approaches will help to personalize interventions because some may be more suitable to patient or caregiver features or resources.

Although behavioral approaches can improve acute mealtime behaviors, less is known about how such approaches change attitudes or associations with the eating context generally, or enjoyment of food, in particular. Children with feeding difficulties and their caregivers have often had extended histories in which eating has been associated with pain[37]; anticipated or experienced dangerous outcomes (eg, exposure to a food allergen); and associations with unpleasant tastes and smells. Negative associations with the social context of eating (eg, parents yelling or nagging) on the part of the child and fatigue on the part of the caregiver are important considerations in the feeding/eating environment. Although the important proximal goal is to increase the mental and physical health of the child, interventions that deliberately attempt to create pleasant associations with the family eating environments and that attempt to decrease caregiver burden and distress are critical components of intervention strategies.[37]

Emerging treatment options for ARFID are currently under development. One psychological treatment being tested at the Massachusetts General Hospital involves cognitive-behavioral therapy for ARFID. This treatment is designed for individuals who are 10 years and older, medically stable, and not using NGT feedings. The treatment consists of 20 to 30 outpatient sessions delivered in an individual or family-supported format and starts with supporting the underweight patient to eat to increase their energy intake resulting in weight restoration. Dietary variety is then increased using structured in-session exposure focusing on the maintaining mechanisms (sensory sensitivity, fear of consequences, or lack of interest in food) of the disorder.[28]

Another novel approach attempts to address eating by helping young children to be less fearful of or less disgusted by bodily and sensory sensations in general, including those involved in eating. Feeling and Body Investigators–ARFID Division uses playful characters (eg, Gassy Gus, Victor Vomit); exercises that intentionally evoke aversive sensations in a playful context (eg, what makes me more nauseous: spinning in a chair for 30 seconds or running in a circle for 30 seconds); and a decision-tree worksheet to help children link body sensations to meaning and actions (I feel gut butterflies: I am nervous, I will go hold someone's hand). The intervention intends to help children be curious investigators of what goes on inside their bodies and what they experience with their senses, rather than fearful. In the context of ARFID, this includes increasing awareness of hunger and fullness and becoming less fearful of vomiting, constipation, and abdominal pain. This intervention has shown preliminary effectiveness in decreasing abdominal pain and anxiety in young children with functional abdominal pain and is being adapted for ARFID.[4]

Box 1 suggests guidelines and future directions for treatment.

Psychiatric medications

There are no evidence-based pharmacologic treatments indicated for the treatment of patients with ARFID. A limited number of reports have described the use of psychotropic medications in both posttraumatic feeding disorders and children and adolescents with ARFID.[39–42] One case series described the use of low-dose olanzapine as an adjunctive treatment to other treatment modalities resulting in reduced anxiety and cognitive features in patients with ARFID.[41] One must consider that patients with ARFID may be better able to metabolize pharmacologic agents because they present

---

Box 1
General guidelines for approaching the management of children with avoidant restrictive food intake disorder

1. Place special emphasis on validating the child and parents' learning history. Given the often extended duration of ARFID, the caregiver/child system may be quite emotionally and physically depleted.

2. Emphasize getting mealtimes back or establishing mealtimes as a safe space. Family mealtimes have often become associated with conflict and distress in families with ARFID. Given the importance of family mealtimes for improving support, communication, manners, teamwork, and other important developmental skills, individuals should consider attempting food challenges at snack times and focusing on consumption of safe foods at mealtimes.

3. If needed, have a comprehensive oral-motor function evaluation so parents and providers feel confident in the types of food that are safe for exposures.

4. Train to confidence in the use of approaches to guarantee safety in the event that exposures trigger an unwanted or potentially dangerous event (eg, accidental exposure to allergen; vomiting; gagging).

5. Facilitate caregiver support.

6. Perform a comprehensive analysis (ie, supervised family meals, or video recordings of mealtimes in the home) to form hypotheses about child and caregiver behaviors that may be reinforcing avoidance of eating and those that increase food approach.

7. Reward the child for engaging in behaviors that increase food approach.

8. Actively supervise and coach parents in the delivery of behavioral management interventions.

9. Consider interventions that address a fear of somatic symptoms in the child, beyond those associated with eating.

Outlined here are suggested guidelines for approaching the management of individuals with ARFID. These are predicated on supporting the underweight and/or growth impaired individual to achieve the rapid restoration of physical health.

---

with higher weights than patients with AN. However, little is known about the benefits and efficacy of these medications in this population, and thus, future randomized, placebo-controlled studies are warranted.

SUMMARY

In the last 5 years, research on ARFID has yielded important new knowledge. Additional epidemiologic studies of ARFID throughout the lifespan are needed. Exploration of risks factors and pathophysiology are critical for developing effective treatment strategies. At present, little is known about how patients with ARFID are best treated across the lifespan. Investigating novel and developmentally-appropriate treatment options and evaluating the efficacy of these options at different levels of care are needed. Furthermore, the development of psychometrically valid measures is essential to help screen for the disorder and evaluate treatment outcomes. More information is needed on ARFID and its associated comorbid medical and mental illnesses, and how this might impact treatment. Other challenging issues confronting the field include the subcategorization of ARFID and the implications of these subcategories on diagnosis and treatment. Emerging evidence holds promise for significantly advancing the understanding of ARFID and the care of patients with this complex disorder.

REFERENCES

1. American Psychiatric Association. Diagnostic and statistical manual of mental disorders: DSM 5. 5th edition. Washington, DC: American Psychiatric Association; 2013.

2. American Psychiatric Association. Diagnostic and statistical manual of mental disorders. 4th edition, text rev. Washington, DC: American Psychiatric Association; 2000.

3. Bryant-Waugh R, Markham L, Kreipe RE, et al. Feeding and eating disorders in childhood. Int J Eat Disord 2010;43(2):98–111.

4. Zucker N, Mauro C, Craske M, et al. Acceptance-based interoceptive exposure for young children with functional abdominal pain. Behav Res Ther 2017;97: 200–12.

5. Mascola AJ, Bryson SW, Agras WS. Picky eating during childhood: a longitudinal study to age 11 years. Eat Behav 2010;11(4):253–7.

6. Pinhas L, Nicholls D, Crosby RD, et al. Classification of childhood onset eating disorders: a latent class analysis. Int J Eat Disord 2017;50(6):657–64.

7. Eddy KT, Thomas JJ, Hastings E, et al. Prevalence of DSM-5 avoidant/restrictive food intake disorder in a pediatric gastroenterology healthcare network. Int J Eat Disord 2015;48(5):464–70.

8. Kurz S, van Dyck Z, Dremmel D, et al. Early-onset restrictive eating disturbances in primary school boys and girls. Eur Child Adolesc Psychiatry 2015;24(7): 779–85.

9. Steen E, Wade TD. Treatment of co-occurring food avoidance and alcohol use disorder in an adult: Possible avoidant restrictive food intake disorder? Int J Eat Disord 2018;51(4):373–7.

10. Lopes R, Melo R, Curral R, et al. A case of choking phobia: towards a conceptual approach. Eat Weight Disord 2014;19(1):125–31.

11. King LA, Urbach JR, Stewart KE. Illness anxiety and avoidant/restrictive food intake disorder: Cognitive-behavioral conceptualization and treatment. Eat Behav 2015;19:106–9.

12. Norris ML, Spettigue W, Hammond NG, et al. Building evidence for the use of descriptive subtypes in youth with avoidant restrictive food intake disorder. Int J Eat Disord 2018;51(2):170–3.

13. Hay P, Mitchison D, Collado AEL, et al. Burden and health-related quality of life of eating disorders, including Avoidant/Restrictive Food Intake Disorder (ARFID), in the Australian population. J Eat Disord 2017;5:21.

14. Kurz S, van Dyck Z, Dremmel D, et al. Variants of early-onset restrictive eating disturbances in middle childhood. Int J Eat Disord 2016;49(1):102–6.

15. Thomas JJ, Lawson EA, Micali N, et al. Avoidant/restrictive food intake disorder: a three-dimensional model of neurobiology with implications for etiology and treatment. Curr Psychiatry Rep 2017;19(8):54.

16. Cooney M, Lieberman M, Guimond T, et al. Clinical and psychological features of children and adolescents diagnosed with avoidant/restrictive food intake disorder in a pediatric tertiary care eating disorder program: a descriptive study. J Eat Disord 2018;6:7.

17. Norris ML, Spettigue WJ, Katzman DK. Update on eating disorders: current perspectives on avoidant/restrictive food intake disorder in children and youth. Neuropsychiatr Dis Treat 2016;12:213–8.

18. Nicely TA, Lane-Loney S, Masciulli E, et al. Prevalence and characteristics of avoidant/restrictive food intake disorder in a cohort of young patients in day treatment for eating disorders. J Eat Disord 2014;2(1):21.

19. Fisher MM, Rosen DS, Ornstein RM, et al. Characteristics of avoidant/restrictive food intake disorder in children and adolescents: a "new disorder" in DSM-5. J Adolesc Health 2014;55(1):49–52.

20. Norris ML, Robinson A, Obeid N, et al. Exploring avoidant/restrictive food intake disorder in eating disordered patients: a descriptive study. Int J Eat Disord 2014; 47(5):495–9.

21. Ornstein RM, Essayli JH, Nicely TA, et al. Treatment of avoidant/restrictive food intake disorder in a cohort of young patients in a partial hospitalization program for eating disorders. Int J Eat Disord 2017;50(9):1067–74.

22. Golden NH, Katzman DK, Sawyer SM, et al. Update on the medical management of eating disorders in adolescents. J Adolesc Health 2015;56(4):370–5.

23. Norris ML, Hiebert JD, Katzman DK. Determining treatment goal weights for children and adolescents with anorexia nervosa. 2018. Available at: https://www.cps.ca/en/documents/position/goal-weights. Accessed April 19, 2018.

24. Zickgraf HF, Franklin ME, Rozin P. Adult picky eaters with symptoms of avoidant/restrictive food intake disorder: comparable distress and comorbidity but different eating behaviors compared to those with disordered eating symptoms. J Eat Disord 2016;4:26.

25. Knaapila A, Silventoinen K, Broms U, et al. Food neophobia in young adults: genetic architecture and relation to personality, pleasantness and use frequency of foods, and body mass index–a twin study. Behav Genet 2011;41(4):512–21.

26. Jaeger SR, Rasmussen MA, Prescott J. Relationships between food neophobia and food intake and preferences: Findings from a sample of New Zealand adults. Appetite 2017;116:410–22.

27. Galloway AT, Fiorito L, Lee Y, et al. Parental pressure, dietary patterns, and weight status among girls who are "picky eaters". J Am Diet Assoc 2005;105(4):541–8.

28. Brigham KS, Manzo LD, Eddy KT, et al. Evaluation and treatment of avoidant/restrictive food intake disorder (ARFID) in adolescents. Curr Pediatr Rep 2018; 6(2):107–13.

29. Zickgraf HF, Ellis JM. Initial validation of the Nine Item Avoidant/Restrictive Food Intake disorder screen (NIAS): a measure of three restrictive eating patterns. Appetite 2018;123:32–42.

30. Forman SF, McKenzie N, Hehn R, et al. Predictors of outcome at 1 year in adolescents with DSM-5 restrictive eating disorders: report of the national eating disorders quality improvement collaborative. J Adolesc Health 2014;55(6):750–6.

31. Strandjord SE, Sieke EH, Richmond M, et al. Avoidant/restrictive food intake disorder: illness and hospital course in patients hospitalized for nutritional insufficiency. J Adolesc Health 2015;57(6):673–8.

32. Nakai Y, Nin K, Noma S, et al. Characteristics of avoidant/restrictive food intake disorder in a cohort of adult patients. Eur Eat Disord Rev 2016;24(6):528–30.

33. Peebles R, Lesser A, Park CC, et al. Outcomes of an inpatient medical nutritional rehabilitation protocol in children and adolescents with eating disorders. J Eat Disord 2017;5:7.

34. Sharp WG, Volkert VM, Scahill L, et al. A systematic review and meta-analysis of intensive multidisciplinary intervention for pediatric feeding disorders: how standard is the standard of care? J Pediatr 2017;181:116–24.e114.

35. Lukens CT, Silverman AH. Systematic review of psychological interventions for pediatric feeding problems. J Pediatr Psychol 2014;39(8):903–17.

36. Sharp WG, Jaquess DL, Morton JF, et al. Pediatric feeding disorders: a quantitative synthesis of treatment outcomes. Clin Child Fam Psychol Rev 2010;13(4): 348–65.
37. Sharp WG, Stubbs KH, Adams H, et al. Intensive, manual-based intervention for pediatric feeding disorders: results from a randomized pilot trial. J Pediatr Gastroenterol Nutr 2016;62(4):658–63.
38. Davis AM, Bruce AS, Mangiaracina C, et al. Moving from tube to oral feeding in medically fragile nonverbal toddlers. J Pediatr Gastroenterol Nutr 2009;49(2): 233–6.
39. Thomas JJ, Brigham KS, Sally ST, et al. Case 18-2017 - an 11-year-old girl with difficulty eating after a choking incident. N Engl J Med 2017;376(24):2377–86.
40. Kardas M, Cermik BB, Ekmekci S, et al. Lorazepam in the treatment of posttraumatic feeding disorder. J Child Adolesc Psychopharmacol 2014;24(5):296–7.
41. Brewerton TD, D'Agostino M. Adjunctive use of olanzapine in the treatment of avoidant restrictive food intake disorder in children and adolescents in an eating disorders program. J Child Adolesc Psychopharmacol 2017;27(10):920–2.
42. Spettigue W, Norris ML, Santos A, et al. Treatment of children and adolescents with avoidant/restrictive food intake disorder: a case series examining the feasibility of family therapy and adjunctive treatments. J Eat Disord 2018;6:20.

Etiological Considerations

Genetics of Eating Disorders
What the Clinician Needs to Know

Cynthia M. Bulik, PhD[a,b,c,]*, Lauren Blake, PhD[d],
Jehannine Austin, PhD, CCGC/CGC[e,f]

KEYWORDS

- Anorexia nervosa • Bulimia nervosa • Binge-eating disorder • Eating disorders
- Genetics • Twin • GWAS • Genetic counseling

KEY POINTS

- Anorexia nervosa, bulimia nervosa, and binge-eating disorder are complex conditions that arise from a combination of genetic and environmental factors.
- Genome-wide association studies of anorexia nervosa have identified specific loci, and genetic correlations implicate both psychiatric and metabolic factors in its origin.
- Patients and families can and do ask about genetic risk for eating disorders and implications for children and other family members.
- Genetic counseling is an important tool to aid families and patients in appraising risk.

STATE OF THE SCIENCE: PSYCHIATRIC GENETICS

Few areas in psychiatry have advanced as rapidly as psychiatric genetics. We can now study the genomes of individuals with and without psychiatric disorders with increasing precision and ever-decreasing costs.[1] Largely through the collaborative efforts of the Psychiatric Genomics Consortium (PGC),[1] our understanding of genetic contributions

Disclosure Statement: C.M. Bulik reports: Shire (grant recipient, Scientific Advisory Board Member), Pearson and Walker (author, royalty recipient), and acknowledges funding from the Swedish Research Council (VR Dnr: 538-2013-8864). L.E. Blake reports: Nothing to disclose. J. Austin reports: Pfizer (investigator initiated, and unrestricted educational grant recipient), W.W. Norton (author).
[a] Department of Psychiatry, UNC Chapel Hill, University of North Carolina, CB 7160, Chapel Hill, NC 27599, USA; [b] Department of Nutrition, University of North Carolina, CB 7400, Chapel Hill, NC 27599, USA; [c] Department of Medical Epidemiology and Biostatistics, Karolinska Institutet, Nobels väg 12A, SE-171 77, Stockholm, Sweden; [d] Department of Human Genetics, University of Chicago, Cummings Life Science Center, 920 East 58th Street, Chicago, IL 60637, USA; [e] Department of Psychiatry, University of British Columbia, Translational Lab Building Room a3-112 – 3rd Floor, 938 West 28th Avenue, Vancouver, British Columbia V5Z 4H4, Canada; [f] Department of Medical Genetics, University of British Columbia, Translational Lab Building Room a3-112 – 3rd Floor, 938 West 28th Avenue, Vancouver, British Columbia V5Z 4H4, Canada
* Corresponding author. Department of Psychiatry, UNC Chapel Hill, University of North Carolina, CB 7160, Chapel Hill, NC 27599
E-mail address: cynthia_bulik@med.unc.edu

to the major psychiatric disorders has burgeoned. The first generation of PGC investigations focused on schizophrenia, major depressive disorder, bipolar disorder, attention-deficit/hyperactivity disorder, and autism spectrum disorder.[2–7] The second generation includes eating disorders, substance use disorders, Tourette syndrome, obsessive-compulsive disorder, and posttraumatic stress disorder.[1] Alzheimer disease and anxiety disorders are provisional groups.[1] The PGC has had impressive successes in both identifying genetic loci associated with specific disorders[4,5,8–15] and advancing our understanding of comorbidity via cross-disorder analyses.[6,16] The challenge for all groups has been to amass adequate sample size to identify a critical number of contributing loci to inform the next steps of explicating biological pathways. Understanding these pathways can ultimately lead to the development of genomically informed therapeutics and allow for increasingly personalized medicine approaches.

Here, the authors present the current state of the science of the Eating Disorders Working Group of the PGC (PGC-ED) and plans for the immediate future.

FAMILY STUDIES, TWIN STUDIES, AND GENOME-WIDE ASSOCIATION STUDIES OF EATING DISORDERS

It is clear that anorexia nervosa (AN), bulimia nervosa (BN), and binge-eating disorder (BED) run in families and are heritable.[17] In the past, the heritability of diseases and disorders had to be estimated indirectly through family or twin studies.[18] Now, we can use genome-wide data to directly estimate heritability.[19–21]

Anorexia Nervosa

AN is familial. Female relatives of individuals with AN are 11 times more likely to develop AN than relatives of individuals without AN.[8] Consistent with the diagnostic flux seen in eating disorders,[22] specific presentations do not breed true in families. For example, the relative risks of full and partial AN syndromes as well as *Diagnostic and Statistical Manual of Mental Disorders*, 4th Edition (DSM-IV) eating disorder not otherwise specified (EDNOS) are elevated in first-degree relatives of individuals with AN and BN.[8,23]

Twin studies have yielded heritability estimates for AN ranging from 0.28 to 0.74.[24–26] The range reflects varying definitions of illness, with more narrow AN definitions associated with higher heritability estimates.[27] Diagnostic transitions between AN and BN are partially accounted for by shared genetic factors, with twin-based genetic correlations ranging between 0.46 and 0.79.[28] Common comorbidities also reflect shared genetic factors with bivariate twin studies of AN with major depression[29] and obsessive-compulsive disorder (OCD)[30] yielding genetic correlations of 0.34 and 0.52, respectively.

Phase I of the PGC-ED was a global collaborative effort including 3495 individuals with AN and nearly 11,000 controls without eating disorder histories from 12 case-control cohorts.[31] The PCG-ED estimated the single nucleotide polymorphism-based heritability of AN to be 0.20, and identified 1 genome-wide significant locus on chromosome 12, that had previously been implicated in type 1 diabetes[32] and rheumatoid arthritis.[33] More broadly, the PCG-ED reported significant genetic correlations between AN and other psychiatric disorders, including schizophrenia, personality traits such as neuroticism, and educational attainment. Of particular interest were significant genetic correlations between AN and metabolic and anthropometric traits, including positive genetic correlations with high-density lipoprotein cholesterol and negative genetic correlations with body mass index (BMI), obesity, fasting insulin, and fasting glucose. Overall, these findings encouraged reconceptualizing AN as both a psychiatric and a metabolic condition.

Critically, increasing sample size will boost power to uncover associations between genetic variants and AN, and to elucidate which biological pathways are important for AN susceptibility. Accordingly, Phase II of the PGC-ED includes more than 16,000 cases and 47,000 controls from 15 countries worldwide. With these data, the PGC-ED is moving closer toward a more comprehensive understanding of how genetic variation contributes to AN risk. The success of the PGC-ED AN genome-wide association study (GWAS) has provided a blueprint for investigating the genetic contributions to other eating disorders.

Bulimia Nervosa

Unfortunately, we know far less about the genetic epidemiology of BN than AN. Individuals with family members diagnosed with BN carry an increased risk of eating disorders and of BN in particular,[8] and the heritability of BN is estimated to be approximately 0.60.[26,28,34,35] AN and BN are strongly genetically correlated (0.46–0.79), as are bulimic behaviors and alcohol misuse (0.33–0.61).[28,36,37] Even though the genetic correlation between AN and BN is high, some specificity may also exist, as co-twins of individuals with bulimic symptoms are at a higher risk for developing BN than AN.[38]

The PGC-ED is actively collecting genetic samples from individuals with BN and will use the GWAS framework to test for genetic variants associated with BN. This initiative will help to elucidate genes and pathways that are shared between BN and AN, and others that are specific to BN.

Binge-Eating Disorder

BED also aggregates in families and is heritable. Few published genetic studies of BED exist, as it has only recently been recognized as an official diagnostic category.[39] Twin-based heritability estimates are between 0.39 and 0.45.[40,41] Significant genetic correlations exist between binge-eating and bulimia symptoms, as well as between binge-eating and alcohol dependence.[36,37,42,43] Obesity and BED are also moderately genetically correlated (0.34).[44] To identify biological pathways involved in BED, the PGC-ED is currently recruiting individuals diagnosed with BED for a GWAS.

Other Eating Disorders

Many of the DSM-5 eating disorders have not yet been the subject of family, twin, or GWA studies. Given the need for large samples, concentrated efforts are needed to make this happen. One approach may be to collect data within countries with health registers or from large health maintenance organizations with electronic databases. However, many countries with health registers use International Classification of Diseases (ICD) rather than DSM codes for disease categorization, meaning that these national resources will not become informative for the new feeding and eating disorders until ICD-11 is launched. Even then, disorder definitions may not map on perfectly to DSM-5.[45] Substantial work will be needed to reconcile these disparities and/or establish additional infrastructure to collect the samples needed.

WHY ARE SUCH LARGE SAMPLE SIZES NECESSARY FOR GENOME-WIDE ASSOCIATION STUDIES?

The most illuminating GWA studies of psychiatric disorders contain tens, or even hundreds of thousands, of cases and controls.[12] The need for large samples is primarily driven by the genetic architecture of complex traits and disorders.[46] These traits are influenced by many genetic variants, but each variant only contributes a small amount to the total phenotypic variation.[47] Increasing the sample size helps to detect variants of small effect while also increasing confidence that any significant variant can be independently replicated.[48]

Findings from the PGC highlight the importance of large numbers of cases and controls.[1] For example, in a schizophrenia GWAS with fewer than 10,000 cases, the genetic variants initially identified failed to replicate.[49] However, in subsequent, larger GWAS for schizophrenia, the PGC identified 108 genetic loci with robust signal.[12] Furthermore, larger sample sizes allow for increased exploration into the mechanisms by which genetic variants influence psychiatric disorder risk, in the cell type(s) important for that disorder.[50–52]

Features of eating disorders, including cross-disorder risk and comorbidities, also necessitate large samples. For example, the high degree of crossover between eating disorders, as well as the high frequency of comorbid disorders (eg, OCD, substance use, anxiety, depression) increases the heterogeneity of the phenotype.[28,36,42,43,53] This means that even more samples are needed to detect true variant-phenotype associations.[54]

Furthermore, genetics may be a viable approach to understand both the role of and the importance of BMI as a diagnostic feature of eating disorders.[38,44] AN is by definition associated with low weight, or substantial weight loss.[39] Atypical AN can be diagnosed in individuals who display all the features of AN except low weight.[39] BED, although commonly associated with overweight or obesity,[38] can and does occur at any weight. As our samples sizes for AN, BN, and BED GWA studies increase, we will be extremely well-positioned to explore how genetic risk for high or low BMI interacts with genetic risk for eating disorders in determining phenotype and perhaps even assist with predicting course of illness and treatment response. For these reasons, the PGC-ED aims to sample more than 100,000 individuals with eating disorders.

WHAT GENOME-WIDE ASSOCIATION STUDIES CAN DELIVER AND WHAT THEY DON'T DELIVER: GENOME-WIDE ASSOCIATION STUDIES TO FUNCTIONALITY, PATHWAYS, THERAPEUTICS

What is the purpose of GWA studies? Historically, in family studies, our goal was to determine whether certain disorders ran in families. The answer to this question was a go/no-go for further exploration of genetic factors via twin and molecular genetic approaches. Twin studies yield heritability estimates, and with caveats, quantify the extent to which familial aggregation reflects genetic factors. To some extent, twin studies provide go/no-go data for GWA studies.

Sullivan and colleagues[1] emphasize that the goals of the PGC are to gain biological, clinical, and therapeutic insights into psychiatric disorders. It is expected that the contribution of individual loci will be small: these are, after all, complex traits. In aggregate, however, many small effect sizes congeal into identifiable pathways that explicate biology. Analyzing the pathways of genome-wide significant variants has confirmed what was previously known about psychiatric disorders and has laid the foundation for new avenues of discovery. For example, the top pathway enriched among schizophrenia GWAS loci, postsynaptic density,[55] was supported by previous copy number variant–based and exome-based studies.[56–58] However, the investigators also found enrichment in the histone H3-K4 methylation pathway.[55] Further exploration of this pathway could shed light on the mechanism(s) underlying environmental risks for schizophrenia occurring early in development.[59–61] We hope for similar insights into eating disorders.

Ultimately targeting pathways (not individual loci of small effect), may have considerable value in the development of pharmacologic interventions. For example, schizophrenia GWAS variants show enrichment for known antipsychotic drugs, including the dopamine D2 receptor (*DRD2*)[62,63] and haloperidol.[64] Additional analyses of these genome-wide significant variants show enrichment for selective calcium channel blockers and antiepileptics, which may be able to be repurposed for schizophrenia treatment.[65] In the same manner, pathways that will be identified in future eating disorder GWA studies may have direct therapeutic implications.

GENES DON'T ACT ALONE

The focus of this review is on genetics; however, none of the work on the genetics of eating disorders precludes the action of the environment on risk. In fact, research on the genetics of eating disorders has thrived because modern technology has made genes more tractable and quantifiable than environmental risk factors. Environmental main effects can occur, and environmental factors can interact with genetic factors in many, often complicated ways. A detailed review of gene-environment interplay in eating disorders can be found in Baker and colleagues.[2]

HOW CAN CLINICIANS USE THIS KNOWLEDGE TO HELP PEOPLE LIVING WITH EATING DISORDERS AND THEIR FAMILIES?

Clinically, individuals with eating disorders and their families and loved ones are deeply interested in the emerging genetic research. In a context in which historically, individuals and their families have been blamed (both overtly and covertly, intentionally and accidentally) for illness,[66–77] genetic explanations for eating disorders hold the attraction of having the potential relieve the burden of blame associated with these conditions.[78,79] Further, genetic findings help validate and legitimize experiences that are often dismissed as "all in the patient's head." However, genetic explanations for conditions like eating disorders are not a panacea: they can inadvertently exacerbate guilt (eg, for "passing on bad genes"), and fear/fatalism (eg, I am doomed to develop an eating disorder because it runs in my family).[79] Further, presenting eating disorders as strictly genetic conditions does not reflect existing knowledge of the complex interplay of genetic and environmental factors.

Providing families with information about causes of illness is, therefore, not a trivial process. The information to be communicated is complex, and its potential emotional ramifications span a broad spectrum.[80,81] Accordingly, clinicians report feeling underprepared to fully engage in discussions about the genetics of psychiatric disorders.[82,83] Families often have pressing questions related to this topic, such as, "Are eating disorders genetic? Is it my fault that I have/my child has an eating disorder? Is the chance that my child will have an eating disorder too great to consider having children? Is there anything I can do to decrease the risk of developing an eating disorder?" In this section, we draw from the field of psychiatric genetic counseling, to provide a framework and resources for clinicians to engage in important conversations around these topics (**Box 1**).

WHAT IS GENETIC COUNSELING?

The need for genetic counseling for people with psychiatric disorders and their families has been discussed in the literature for years,[84–90] with empirical studies emerging in the past decade.[91–98] Even in the absence of genetic testing, genetic counseling to help people make meaning of genetic information from their family history can lead to important outcomes, including improved knowledge, more accurate understanding of risk,[94] and increased empowerment and self-efficacy.[93] To date there are, to our

---

Box 1
What is genetic counseling

Though often thought of as being an activity (ie, a conversation any health care provider might have about genetic testing or risk for children), genetic counseling is a professional discipline in its own right. The first MSc level training program was established at Sarah Lawrence College in the 1960s, and there are currently ~4000 board-certified genetic counselors practicing in North America.[108] Genetic counseling is not dependent on genetic testing, is not a purely educational or informational interaction, and is not solely focused on conversations about risks for family members or pregnancy. Instead genetic counseling is the process of helping people to "understand and adapt to the medical psychological and familial implications of genetic contributions to disease."[109] The profession is founded on a patient-centered counseling model, and the principle of promoting and supporting patient autonomy is fundamental.[81] A key focus of genetic counseling is to uncover and address any guilt, shame, stigma, blame, or fear that may relate specifically to the patient/family's explanation for cause of the condition in the family. Genetic counselors also take a personalized approach to helping patients to make decisions (when applicable, eg, concerning childbearing) that are best for them, based on their own values, practicalities, and priorities. Genetic counseling differs in important ways from the group-based psychoeducation that often occurs in psychiatric settings. Although there is some overlap in the roles of genetic counselors and psychiatrists (especially in terms of uncovering and addressing emotions), the scope for genetic counselors is limited to addressing these issues as they relate to people's explanations for cause of illness. Further, the relationship that a psychiatrist has with a patient is typically longer term, whereas genetic counseling typically is limited to 1 to 2 appointments.[93] Genetic counseling can be delivered to an individual patient alone, to various configurations of the patient and family members, to couples, or family members without the patient present.

---

knowledge, no empirical studies specifically exploring genetic counseling in eating disorders.

Eating disorder clinicians may not be inclined to develop the expertise necessary to engage in discussions about genetics with their patients. Such a situation is ideal for interdisciplinary collaboration: clinicians can partner with genetic counselors to provide these services to families (www.findageneticcounselor.com). For clinicians who wish to engage with families around genetic topics, we provide a brief guide (see Ref.[80] for more comprehensive guidelines).

GETTING STARTED

A detailed 3-generation psychiatric history is a key tool for the genetic counseling process.[99] It can be used as a starting point for discussions about explanations for cause of illness, and for conversations about risk for family members (if requested). This detailed history can be taken before (eg, via telephone)[100] or during sessions focused on genetic topics.

Genetic counseling involves a bi-directional exchange of information between clinician and patient, in the context of a psychotherapeutically oriented encounter.[101] The clinician or genetic counselor should focus on identifying, uncovering, and addressing emotions that may be driving the patient's questions and assumptions. Genetic counseling sessions (either by a trained genetic counselor or a clinician in this role) begin with an initial contracting process, exploring the patient's questions and concerns, setting expectations around duration of encounter, etc. Then, the detailed 3-generation psychiatric history picture is used to initiate a conversation about the patient's existing explanation for cause of illness.[102] This is important, because if new information does not account for (reinforce or challenge) existing explanations, it can easily be dismissed as irrelevant to an individual's unique situation.[103]

DISCUSSING GENETIC RESEARCH AND THE ETIOLOGY OF EATING DISORDERS

Typically, patients and families are not interested in, and do not need to know, names of specific genetic variants. Seeking information about causes of conditions like eating disorders is rarely a purely intellectual enterprise; even detailed questions about specific variants are often driven by fear, guilt, or a need for control or certainty. It is crucial to convey the following to families:

- Eating disorders arise from the combined effects of genes and environment (or experiences).
- We do not typically inherit mental illness, but we can inherit a vulnerability to mental illness.
- There is no known single factor that is necessary and sufficient to cause eating disorders.

No statements around these issues are neutral; their valence is subjective. Therefore, it is important to address the emotions attached to these issues, which may range from intense relief ("Oh thank goodness; it's not my fault!") to deep worry ("How vulnerable am I?/Does this mean that [experience that I feel responsible for] is why I have this condition...IS it my fault?"), or guilt ("Did this happen because I passed on bad genes?").

Visual counseling aids (like the "Jar model,"[80] which applies the concept of different shapes for genetic and environmental vulnerability factors filling a jar, available at nsgc.org) can pictorially represent how illness occurs. A key message that can be profound and de-stigmatizing is that we all have some genetic vulnerability to eating disorders.[31] The family history picture can be used to personalize the discussion about etiology and illustrate how genes and experiences may have co-contributed for individuals in their family. When multiple psychiatric and metabolic disorders aggregate in the family, it can also be useful for families to have a discussion, based on the family history picture, about how GWA studies demonstrate that genetic vulnerability can be shared across these different conditions.[20,31] Clarifying the etiology of eating disorders can be used as a framework for understanding not just how people develop illness, but to contextualize what might be done to mitigate risk, or to support recovery (as described in Ref.[80]).

IMPLICATIONS OF ETIOLOGY: DISCUSSING TREATMENTS FOR AND RECOVERY FROM EATING DISORDERS

Clarifying the etiology of eating disorders can also be used as a framework for understanding what might be done to mitigate risk, or to support recovery. The clinician should ensure that the patient and/or family understands (again using visual aids) that we cannot change our genetic vulnerability to eating disorders, but we may be able to manage some aspects of how our environment shapes our risk. It is important to ensure that the patient and/or family understands that we cannot categorically prevent development of an eating disorder, but we may be able to protect mental health. For example, in general, social support, adequate regular sleep, good-quality regular nutrition, exercise (in moderation), and developing effective stress management techniques can all be beneficial to general mental health,[104–106] as well as other activities that may be effective for some individuals too (eg, spending time with a pet, reading fiction). The clinician should work to help the patient and/or family identify other strategies, and to acknowledge the guilt that can accompany failing to engage in all of these activities all the time, perfectly. The goal is to simply do what we can, celebrate those achievements, and practice self-compassion, because perfection is not possible.

For parents of children with eating disorders, creating an environment in which discussing mental health is not taboo, and where good communication and support are prioritized, and mental health self-care is modeled can only help. It is very important to convey to parents that perfect parenting does not exist. No parent has the power to categorically prevent illness.

DISCUSSING RISK FOR EATING DISORDERS IN THE FAMILY

Communicating about risk is not a necessary component of the genetic counseling interaction.[107] Even when patients state that the reason for seeking counseling is to understand the chances of family members developing an eating disorder, it is beneficial to begin with a discussion of etiology and the implications for treatment and recovery. This exchange serves as a framework for any discussion about probabilities. Once the patient is satisfied with her or his understanding of these topics, then reassess their interest in discussing specific probabilities. After addressing these topics, approximately 20% of patients change their mind about discussing specific probabilities.[107] Sometimes, understanding that illness is not inevitable, and that some strategies exist that can protect mental health is enough. Indeed, those who veer away from seeking concrete numbers tend to have better outcomes in genetic counseling.[107] When a patient or family does desire a discussion of risk, it should be approached carefully, as outlined in **Table 1**.

Table 1
Process for engaging patients with eating disorders and/or their family members in discussion about risk for recurrence

Step 1: Assess expectations[a]	Ask the patient/family if they have a sense of what the chance might be and what informed their perception.
Step 2: Assess probability	Any numbers provided should not be based solely on empirical data. Clinical judgment is required to modify (as described in Ref.[110]) chances for recurrence that have been determined in empirical studies according to the 3-generation targeted family history.
Step 3: Provide numbers	Although it may be tempting to simply offer a qualitative assessment of the risk, rather than numbers, this is inadvisable and can lead to problematic clinical miscommunication.[111] Specifically, perception of risk is subjective, and therefore what is considered "a high chance" by one individual may be perceived as "low" by another.[112] Framing and simplicity are important when providing numbers for example, "there is a 10% or 1 in 10 chance that your child would develop [condition X].[112] That's the same as saying there is a 90% chance of a 9 in 10 chance that they will not develop [condition X]."
Step 4: Contextualize	Contextualize the numbers provided in terms of general population figures (eg, "everyone has some chance of developing [condition X], in the general population the chance to develop it is y% or 1 in z").
Step 5: Check in	Ask the patient and/or family to reflect on their reactions to the numbers.

[a] Consider who requests a discussion of risk. Chances for a child to develop an eating disorder should not be discussed with anyone other than the child or the child's parent/guardian.
Data from Ryan J, Virani A, Austin JC. Ethical issues associated with genetic counseling in the context of adolescent psychiatry. Appl Transl Genom 2015;5:23–9.

PRENATAL GENETIC COUNSELING FOR EATING DISORDERS: A SPECIAL NOTE

It can be helpful for individuals with eating disorders who are concerned about whether they should have children to explore perceptions of and emotions around the causes of and risk for eating disorders. In this context, it is particularly important to ensure clarity around the following:

- It is not a foregone conclusion that a child will develop an eating disorder, even if *both* parents have diagnoses.
- There are things that can be done to protect mental health, but there is no such thing as perfect parenting, and no way to definitively prevent mental illness.

Careful discussion of these issues and fears around hypervigilance, living with uncertainty, and relapse in the perinatal period can help people to arrive at decisions about how to move forward, given their values, priorities, and practical circumstances (for a deeper discussion, see Ref.[102]).

SUMMARY

Genetic research in eating disorders is accelerating rapidly and we expect significant new findings for AN, BN, and BED to emerge in the coming years. Concerted efforts must also be made to extend genetic research to other eating disorder presentations, such as avoidant and restrictive food-intake disorder, Other specified feeding or eating disorder, and atypical AN. As lay awareness of genetic factors in eating disorders grows, so too does the need for support for patients and families to contextualize and process this biological information. Clinicians and genetic counselors can both play important roles in this process. The discussion provided here can equip clinicians who are motivated to engage in conversations around these topics with the basics for meaningful engagement. However, this is a domain in which interdisciplinary collaboration between genetic counselors and physicians may be an optimal strategy for supporting patients and their families in their process of gaining new understandings and making sense of the complex role of genetics in eating disorders.

REFERENCES

1. Sullivan PF, Agrawal A, Bulik CM, et al. Psychiatric genomics: an update and an agenda. Am J Psychiatry 2018;175:15–27.
2. Baker JH, Schaumberg K, Munn-Chernoff MA. Genetics of anorexia nervosa. Curr Psychiatry Rep 2017;19:84.
3. Major Depressive Disorder Working Group of the Psychiatric Genomics Consortium, Ripke S, Wray NR, Lewis CM, et al. A mega-analysis of genome-wide association studies for major depressive disorder. Mol Psychiatry 2013;18: 497–511.
4. Neale BM, Medland SE, Ripke S, et al. Meta-analysis of genome-wide association studies of attention-deficit/hyperactivity disorder. J Am Acad Child Adolesc Psychiatry 2010;49:884–97.
5. Autism Spectrum Disorders Working Group of The Psychiatric Genomics Consortium. Meta-analysis of GWAS of over 16,000 individuals with autism spectrum disorder highlights a novel locus at 10q24.32 and a significant overlap with schizophrenia. Mol Autism 2017;8:21.
6. Cross-Disorder Group of the Psychiatric Genomics Consortium. Identification of risk loci with shared effects on five major psychiatric disorders: a genome-wide analysis. Lancet 2013;381:1371–9.
7. Schizophrenia Psychiatric Genome-Wide Association Study Consortium. Genome-wide association study identifies five new schizophrenia loci. Nat Genet 2011;43:969–76.

8. Strober M, Freeman R, Lampert C, et al. Controlled family study of anorexia nervosa and bulimia nervosa: evidence of shared liability and transmission of partial syndromes. Am J Psychiatry 2000;157:393–401.

9. Scharf JM, Yu D, Mathews CA, et al. Genome-wide association study of Tourette's syndrome. Mol Psychiatry 2013;18:721–8.

10. Mattheisen M, Samuels JF, Wang Y, et al. Genome-wide association study in obsessive-compulsive disorder: results from the OCGAS. Mol Psychiatry 2015;20:337–44.

11. Duncan LE, Ratanatharathorn A, Aiello AE, et al. Largest GWAS of PTSD (N=20 070) yields genetic overlap with schizophrenia and sex differences in heritability. Mol Psychiatry 2018;23:666–73.

12. Schizophrenia Working Group of the Psychiatric Genomics Consortium. Biological insights from 108 schizophrenia-associated genetic loci. Nature 2014;511: 421–7.

13. Wray NR, Ripke S, Mattheisen M, et al. Genome-wide association analyses identify 44 risk variants and refine the genetic architecture of major depression. Nat Genet 2018;50:668–81.

14. Stahl E, Breen G, Forstner A, et al. Genomewide association study identifies 30 loci associated with bipolar disorder. bioRxiv 2018;173062. https://doi.org/10.1101/173062.

15. Walters R, Adams M, Adkins A. Trans-ancestral GWAS of alcohol dependence reveals common genetic underpinnings with psychiatric disorders. bioRxiv 2018;257311. https://doi.org/10.1101/257311.

16. Bulik-Sullivan BK, Loh PR, Finucane HK, et al. LD score regression distinguishes confounding from polygenicity in genome-wide association studies. Nat Genet 2015;47:291–5.

17. Yilmaz Z, Hardaway JA, Bulik CM. Genetics and epigenetics of eating disorders. Adv Genomics Genet 2015;5:131–50.

18. Visscher PM, Hill WG, Wray NR. Heritability in the genomics era—concepts and misconceptions. Nat Rev Genet 2008;9:255–66.

19. Yang J, Lee SH, Goddard ME, et al. GCTA: a tool for genome-wide complex trait analysis. Am J Hum Genet 2011;88:76–82.

20. Bulik-Sullivan B, Finucane HK, Anttila V, et al. An atlas of genetic correlations across human diseases and traits. Nat Genet 2015;47:1236–41.

21. Psychiatric GWAS Consortium Steering Committee. A framework for interpreting genome-wide association studies of psychiatric disorders. Mol Psychiatry 2009; 14:10–7.

22. Schaumberg K, Jangmo A, Thornton L, et al. Patterns of diagnostic flux in eating disorders: a longitudinal population study in Sweden. Psychol Med 2018. [Epub ahead of print].

23. Lilenfeld LR, Kaye WH, Greeno CG, et al. A controlled family study of anorexia nervosa and bulimia nervosa: psychiatric disorders in first-degree relatives and effects of proband comorbidity. Arch Gen Psychiatry 1998;55:603–10.

24. Bulik CM, Sullivan PF, Tozzi F, et al. Prevalence, heritability and prospective risk factors for anorexia nervosa. Arch Gen Psychiatry 2006;63:305–12.

25. Klump KL, Miller KB, Keel PK, et al. Genetic and environmental influences on anorexia nervosa syndromes in a population-based twin sample. Psychol Med 2001;31:737–40.

26. Kortegaard LS, Hoerder K, Joergensen J, et al. A preliminary population-based twin study of self-reported eating disorder. Psychol Med 2001;31:361–5.

27. Dellava JE, Thornton LM, Lichtenstein P, et al. Impact of broadening definitions of anorexia nervosa on sample characteristics. J Psychiatr Res 2011;45:691–8.

28. Bulik CM, Thornton LM, Root TL, et al. Understanding the relation between anorexia nervosa and bulimia nervosa in a Swedish national twin sample. Biol Psychiatry 2010;67:71–7.

29. Wade TD, Bulik CM, Neale M, et al. Anorexia nervosa and major depression: shared genetic and environmental risk factors. Am J Psychiatry 2000;157: 469–71.

30. Cederlöf M, Thornton LM, Baker JH, et al. Etiological overlap between obsessive-compulsive disorder and anorexia nervosa: a longitudinal cohort, family and twin study. World Psychiatry 2015;14:333–8.

31. Duncan L, Yilmaz Z, Gaspar H, et al. Significant locus and metabolic genetic correlations revealed in genome-wide association study of anorexia nervosa. Am J Psychiatry 2017;174:850–8.

32. Barrett JC, Clayton DG, Concannon P, et al. Genome-wide association study and meta-analysis find that over 40 loci affect risk of type 1 diabetes. Nat Genet 2009;41:703–7.

33. Okada Y, Wu D, Trynka G, et al. Genetics of rheumatoid arthritis contributes to biology and drug discovery. Nature 2014;506:376–81.

34. Bulik CM, Sullivan PF, Kendler KS. Heritability of binge-eating and broadly defined bulimia nervosa. Biol Psychiatry 1998;44:1210–8.

35. Trace SE, Thornton LM, Baker JH, et al. A behavioral-genetic investigation of bulimia nervosa and its relationship with alcohol use disorder. Psychiatry Res 2013;208:232–7.

36. Slane JD, Burt SA, Klump KL. Bulimic behaviors and alcohol use: shared genetic influences. Behav Genet 2012;42:603–13.

37. Munn-Chernoff MA, Grant JD, Agrawal A, et al. Genetic overlap between alcohol use disorder and bulimic behaviors in European American and African American women. Drug Alcohol Depend 2015;153:335–40.

38. Bulik CM, Sullivan PF, Kendler KS. An empirical study of the classification of eating disorders. Am J Psychiatry 2000;157:886–95.

39. American Psychiatric Association. Diagnostic and statistical manual of mental disorders. 5th edition. Arlington (VA): American Psychiatric Association Publishing; 2013.

40. Javaras KN, Laird NM, Reichborn-Kjennerud T, et al. Familiality and heritability of binge eating disorder: results of a case-control family study and a twin study. Int J Eat Disord 2008;41:174–9.

41. Mitchell KS, Neale MC, Bulik CM, et al. Binge eating disorder: a symptom-level investigation of genetic and environmental influences on liability. Psychol Med 2010;40:1899–906.

42. Munn-Chernoff MA, Baker JH. A primer on the genetics of comorbid eating disorders and substance use disorders. Eur Eat Disord Rev 2016;24:91–100.

43. Munn-Chernoff MA, Duncan AE, Grant JD, et al. A twin study of alcohol dependence, binge eating, and compensatory behaviors. J Stud Alcohol Drugs 2013; 74:664–73.

44. Bulik CM, Sullivan PF, Kendler KS. Genetic and environmental contributions to obesity and binge eating. Int J Eat Disord 2003;33:293–8.

45. World Health Organization. Feeding or eating disorders. 2018. Available at: https://icd.who.int/browse11/l-m/en#/http%3a%2f%2fid.who.int%2ficd%2fentity %2f1412387537. Accessed July 8, 2018.

46. Sullivan PF, Daly MJ, O'Donovan M. Genetic architectures of psychiatric disorders: the emerging picture and its implications. Nat Rev Genet 2012;13:537–51.
47. Fu W, O'Connor TD, Akey JM. Genetic architecture of quantitative traits and complex diseases. Curr Opin Genet Dev 2013;23:678–83.
48. Kraft P, Zeggini E, Ioannidis JP. Replication in genome-wide association studies. Stat Sci 2009;24:561–73.
49. International Schizophrenia Consortium, Purcell SM, Wray NR, Stone JL, et al. Common polygenic variation contributes to risk of schizophrenia and bipolar disorder. Nature 2009;460:748–52.
50. Gusev A, Mancuso N, Won H, et al. Transcriptome-wide association study of schizophrenia and chromatin activity yields mechanistic disease insights. Nat Genet 2018;50:538–48.
51. Park Y, Sarkar A, Bhutani K, et al. Multi-tissue polygenic models for transcriptome-wide association studies. bioRxiv 2017;107623. https://doi.org/10.1101/107623.
52. Fromer M, Roussos P, Sieberts SK, et al. Gene expression elucidates functional impact of polygenic risk for schizophrenia. Nat Neurosci 2016;19:1442–53.
53. Yilmaz Z, Halvorsen M, Bryois J, et al. Examination of the shared genetic basis of anorexia nervosa and obsessive-compulsive disorder. Mol Psychiatry 2018. [Epub ahead of print].
54. Manchia M, Cullis J, Turecki G, et al. The impact of phenotypic and genetic heterogeneity on results of genome wide association studies of complex diseases. PLoS One 2013;8:e76295.
55. Network and Pathway Analysis Subgroup of Psychiatric Genomics Consortium. Psychiatric genome-wide association study analyses implicate neuronal, immune and histone pathways. Nat Neurosci 2015;18:199–209.
56. Kirov G, Pocklington AJ, Holmans P, et al. De novo CNV analysis implicates specific abnormalities of postsynaptic signalling complexes in the pathogenesis of schizophrenia. Mol Psychiatry 2012;17:142–53.
57. Purcell SM, Moran JL, Fromer M, et al. A polygenic burden of rare disruptive mutations in schizophrenia. Nature 2014;506:185–90.
58. Fromer M, Pocklington AJ, Kavanagh DH, et al. De novo mutations in schizophrenia implicate synaptic networks. Nature 2014;506:179–84.
59. Susser E, St Clair D, He L. Latent effects of prenatal malnutrition on adult health: the example of schizophrenia. Ann N Y Acad Sci 2008;1136:185–92.
60. Heijmans BT, Tobi EW, Lumey LH, et al. The epigenome: archive of the prenatal environment. Epigenetics 2009;4:526–31.
61. Huang HS, Matevossian A, Whittle C, et al. Prefrontal dysfunction in schizophrenia involves mixed-lineage leukemia 1-regulated histone methylation at GABAergic gene promoters. J Neurosci 2007;27:11254–62.
62. Lencz T, Malhotra AK. Targeting the schizophrenia genome: a fast track strategy from GWAS to clinic. Mol Psychiatry 2015;20:820–6.
63. Kapur S, Mamo D. Half a century of antipsychotics and still a central role for dopamine D2 receptors. Prog Neuropsychopharmacol Biol Psychiatry 2003;27:1081–90.
64. Kim Y, Giusti-Rodriguez P, Crowley JJ, et al. Comparative genomic evidence for the involvement of schizophrenia risk genes in antipsychotic effects. Mol Psychiatry 2018;23:708–12.
65. Gaspar HA, Breen G. Pathways analyses of schizophrenia GWAS focusing on known and novel drug targets. bioRxiv 2017;091264. https://doi.org/10.1101/091264.

66. Crisafulli MA, Von Holle A, Bulik CM. Attitudes towards anorexia nervosa: the impact of framing on blame and stigma. Int J Eat Disord 2008;41:333–9.
67. Roehrig JP, McLean CP. A comparison of stigma toward eating disorders versus depression. Int J Eat Disord 2010;43:671–4.
68. Ebneter DS, Latner JD. Stigmatizing attitudes differ across mental health disorders: a comparison of stigma across eating disorders, obesity, and major depressive disorder. J Nerv Ment Dis 2013;201:281–5.
69. Bowlby J. Maternal care and mental health. Bull World Health Organ 1951;3: 355–533.
70. Dixon MJ, King S, Stip E, et al. Continuous performance test differences among schizophrenic out-patients living in high and low expressed emotion environments. Psychol Med 2000;30:1141–53.
71. Campbell K, Peebles R. Eating disorders in children and adolescents: state of the art review. Pediatrics 2014;134:582–92.
72. Eisler I. The empirical and theoretical base of family therapy and multiple family day therapy for adolescent anorexia nervosa. J Fam Ther 2005;27:104–31.
73. Larsen PS, Strandberg-Larsen K, Micali N, et al. Parental and child characteristics related to early-onset disordered eating: a systematic review. Harv Rev Psychiatry 2015;23:395–412.
74. le Grange D, Lock J, Loeb K, et al. Academy for eating disorders position paper: the role of the family in eating disorders. Int J Eat Disord 2010;43:1–5.
75. Strober M, Humphrey LL. Familial contributions to the etiology and course of anorexia nervosa and bulimia. J Consult Clin Psychol 1987;55:654–9.
76. Schaumberg K, Welch E, Breithaupt L, et al. The science behind the Academy for Eating Disorders' nine truths about eating disorders. Eur Eat Disord Rev 2017;25:432–50.
77. Yager J. Family issues in the pathogenesis of anorexia nervosa. Psychosom Med 1982;44:43–60.
78. Phelan JC. Genetic bases of mental illness—a cure for stigma? Trends Neurosci 2002;25:430–1.
79. Austin JC, Honer WG. The potential impact of genetic counseling for mental illness. Clin Genet 2005;67:134–42.
80. Peay H, Austin J. How to talk to families about genetics and psychiatric disorders. 1st edition. New York: W.W. Norton & Company; 2011.
81. Veach PM, Bartels DM, Leroy BS. Coming full circle: a reciprocal-engagement model of genetic counseling practice. J Genet Couns 2007;16:713–28.
82. Hoop JG, Roberts LW, Hammond KAG, et al. Psychiatrists' attitudes, knowledge, and experience regarding genetics: a preliminary study. Genet Med 2008;10:439.
83. Zhou YZ, Wilde A, Meiser B, et al. Attitudes of medical genetics practitioners and psychiatrists toward communicating with patients about genetic risk for psychiatric disorders. Psychiatr Genet 2014;24:94–101.
84. Stancer HC, Wagener DK. Genetic counselling: its need in psychiatry and the directions it gives for future research. Can J Psychiatry 1984;29:289–94.
85. Papadimitriou GN, Dikeos DG. How does recent knowledge on the heredity of schizophrenia affect genetic counseling? Curr Psychiatry Rep 2003;5:239–40.
86. Kumar P. Genetic counselling in family planning. Antiseptic 1968;65(11):831–4.
87. Hodgkinson KA, Murphy J, O'Neill S, et al. Genetic counselling for schizophrenia in the era of molecular genetics. Can J Psychiatry 2001;46:123–30.
88. Tsuang DW, Faraone SV, Tsuang MT. Genetic counseling for psychiatric disorders. Curr Psychiatry Rep 2001;3:138–43.

89. Reveley A. Genetic counselling for schizophrenia. Br J Psychiatry 1985;147: 107–12.
90. Finn CT, Smoller JW. Genetic counseling in psychiatry. Harv Rev Psychiatry 2006;14:109–21.
91. Austin JC, Honer WG. Psychiatric genetic counselling for parents of individuals affected with psychotic disorders: a pilot study. Early Interv Psychiatry 2008;2: 80–9.
92. Hippman C, Lohn Z, Ringrose A, et al. "Nothing is absolute in life": understanding uncertainty in the context of psychiatric genetic counseling from the perspective of those with serious mental illness. J Genet Couns 2013;22: 625–32.
93. Inglis A, Koehn D, McGillivray B, et al. Evaluating a unique, specialist psychiatric genetic counseling clinic: uptake and impact. Clin Genet 2015;87:218–24.
94. Hippman C, Ringrose A, Inglis A, et al. A pilot randomized clinical trial evaluating the impact of genetic counseling for serious mental illnesses. J Clin Psychiatry 2016;77:e190–8.
95. Leach E, Morris E, White HJ, et al. How do physicians decide to refer their patients for psychiatric genetic counseling? A qualitative study of physicians' practice. J Genet Couns 2016;25:1235–42.
96. Moldovan R, Pintea S, Austin J. The efficacy of genetic counseling for psychiatric disorders: a meta-analysis. J Genet Couns 2017;26:1341–7.
97. Costain G, Esplen MJ, Toner B, et al. Evaluating genetic counseling for individuals with schizophrenia in the molecular age. Schizophr Bull 2014;40:78–87.
98. Costain G, Esplen MJ, Toner B, et al. Evaluating genetic counseling for family members of individuals with schizophrenia in the molecular age. Schizophr Bull 2014;40:88–99.
99. Bennett RL, French KS, Resta RG, et al. Standardized human pedigree nomenclature: update and assessment of the recommendations of the National Society of Genetic Counselors. J Genet Couns 2008;17:424–33.
100. Slomp C, Morris E, Inglis A, et al. Patient outcomes of genetic counseling: assessing the impact of different approaches to family history collection. Clin Genet 2018;93:830–6.
101. Austin J, Semaka A, Hadjipavlou G. Conceptualizing genetic counseling as psychotherapy in the era of genomic medicine. J Genet Couns 2014;23:903–9.
102. Inglis A, Morris E, Austin J. Prenatal genetic counselling for psychiatric disorders. Prenat Diagn 2017;37:6–13.
103. Skirton H, Eiser C. Discovering and addressing the client's lay construct of genetic disease: an important aspect of genetic healthcare? Res Theory Nurs Pract 2003;17:339–52.
104. Nowlin-Finch NL, Altshuler LL, Szuba MP, et al. Rapid resolution of first episodes of mania: sleep related? J Clin Psychiatry 1994;55:26–9.
105. Peet M, Horrobin DF. A dose-ranging study of the effects of ethyl-eicosapentaenoate in patients with ongoing depression despite apparently adequate treatment with standard drugs. Arch Gen Psychiatry 2002;59:913–9.
106. Scheewe TW, Backx FJ, Takken T, et al. Exercise therapy improves mental and physical health in schizophrenia: a randomised controlled trial. Acta Psychiatr Scand 2013;127:464–73.
107. Borle K, Morris E, Inglis A, et al. Risk communication in genetic counseling: exploring uptake and perception of recurrence numbers, and their impact on patient outcomes. Clin Genet 2018;94(2):239–45.

108. Ormond KE, Laurino MY, Barlow-Stewart K, et al. Genetic counseling globally: Where are we now? Am J Med Genet C Semin Med Genet 2018;178:98–107.
109. National Society of Genetic Counselors' Definition Task Force, Resta R, Biesecker BB, Bennett RL, et al. A new definition of genetic counseling: National Society of Genetic Counselors' task force report. J Genet Couns 2006;15:77–83.
110. Austin JC, Palmer CG, Rosen-Sheidley B, et al. Psychiatric disorders in clinical genetics II: individualizing recurrence risks. J Genet Couns 2008;17:18–29.
111. Austin JC, Hippman C, Honer WG. Descriptive and numeric estimation of risk for psychotic disorders among affected individuals and relatives: implications for clinical practice. Psychiatry Res 2012;196:52–6.
112. Austin JC. Re-conceptualizing risk in genetic counseling: implications for clinical practice. J Genet Couns 2010;19:228–34.

Cognitive Neuroscience of Eating Disorders

Joanna E. Steinglass, MD[a],*, Laura A. Berner, PhD[b], Evelyn Attia, MD[a]

KEYWORDS

- Eating disorders • Neuroscience • Anorexia nervosa • Bulimia nervosa
- Cognitive neuroscience • Neurobiology

KEY POINTS

- Cognitive neuroscience offers research approaches that can test hypotheses about the link between maladaptive eating behavior and underlying neural systems, thereby helping to further our understanding of eating disorders.
- Reward-focused approaches have identified reward processing and learning abnormalities in anorexia nervosa, which have been less studied in bulimia nervosa.
- Control-focused approaches suggest corticostriatal abnormalities in bulimia nervosa associated with dysfunction in cognitive and behavioral control.
- Decision-making approaches show that the neural mechanisms of food choice among patients with anorexia nervosa differ from healthy individuals.

INTRODUCTION

Eating disorders are characterized by a combination of disturbances in body image and maladaptive eating behaviors. The neural mechanisms remain unclear, and perhaps less clear than for other psychiatric illnesses with a similar public health impact. Early approaches to understanding the neurobiology underlying these complex disorders focused on neurotransmitters and identified differences in the presence and metabolism of dopamine and serotonin.[1,2] As neuroscience and neuroimaging have advanced, it has become increasingly possible to examine the neural systems that govern human behavior. These advances can be leveraged in psychiatry to link brain activity with maladaptive behavior. One perspective focuses on neural systems that have been well-characterized and tests whether these systems function normally in the setting of illness—a bottom-up approach. An alternative perspective starts with

Disclosures: J.E. Steinglass and E. Attia receive royalties from UpToDate.
a Department of Psychiatry, New York State Psychiatric Institute, Columbia University Irving Medical Center, 1051 Riverside Drive, Unit 98, New York, NY 10032, USA; b Department of Psychiatry, University of California, San Diego, Eating Disorders Center for Treatment and Research, 4510 Executive Drive, Suite 330, San Diego, CA 92121, USA
* Corresponding author.
E-mail address: Js1124@cumc.columbia.edu

psych.theclinics.com

Abbreviations	
ACC	Anterior cingulate cortex
AN	Anorexia nervosa
BN	Bulimia nervosa
dlPFC	Dorsolateral PFC
fMRI	Functional MRI
OFC	Orbitofrontal cortex
PFC	Prefrontal cortex

clinical phenomena and abnormal behavior and tests hypotheses about neural under-pinnings—a top-down approach (**Fig. 1**). Both methods use brain–behavior models to develop and systematically test hypotheses.

In this review, the authors describe the existing data on neural mechanisms of eating disorders, focusing on 3 areas that suggest paths forward: reward, behavioral and cognitive control, and decision making. To date, the majority of research in these areas comes from anorexia nervosa (AN) and bulimia nervosa (BN); therefore, this review focuses on the neural mechanisms for these disorders.

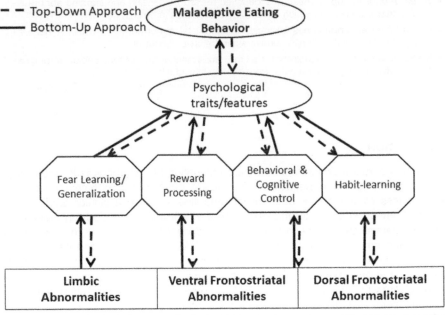

Fig. 1. Modeling the links between brain and behavior to create specific testable hypotheses. Maladaptive eating behavior consists of food avoidance and rigid dieting practices in anorexia nervosa (AN) and in bulimia nervosa (BN), and out-of-control binge eating and compensatory behaviors in BN and the binge-eating/purging subtype of AN. These maladaptive behaviors are associated with numerous psychological traits, such as high anxiety and high obsessionality. These traits, in turn, are associated with specific neurocognitive processes that are the behavioral output associated with neural circuits. Fear learning processes are related to limbic circuits and are associated with anxiety and avoidance behaviors. Reward processing and learning are associated with ventral frontostriatal circuits and relate to hedonic processes as well as the development of learned behaviors (perhaps including dieting). Control processes and habit learning are associated with dorsal frontostriatal circuits and are related to disinhibition and obsessionality, which are also related to eating disordered behaviors.

Each of these areas includes a range of cognitive–behavioral processes and associated neural systems. Reward has been parsed into hedonic value (or liking), motivational salience (or wanting), and reinforcement learning.[3,4] The reward system in the brain is composed of the midbrain/ventral tegmental area, ventral striatum (including the nucleus accumbens), medial prefrontal cortex (prefrontal cortex), and orbitofrontal cortex (OFC). Reward-centered models in AN have hypothesized both hyporesponsiveness to reward and aberrant reward attribution (ie, positive stimuli become aversive and vice versa, such that hunger becomes rewarding).[5] In BN, theoretic models posit that increased expectancy of reward, but decreased experienced reward from eating may contribute to maladaptive behavior patterns.[6]

Behavioral and cognitive control processes include response inhibition (or inhibitory control), attentional control, and cognitive flexibility. These processes recruit overlapping frontostriatal, cinguloopercular, and frontoparietal networks[7–10]; the PFC are generally viewed as the central executors of control.[11,12] In AN, patterns of restrictive eating are interpreted as extremes of self-control. BN is associated with impulsivity and the tendency to act rashly in the context of negative emotion.[13] Such observations raise questions about the functioning of neural systems associated with behavioral and cognitive control across eating disorders.[14]

Decision making can be considered an end-result of reward and control processes. In cognitive neuroscience, this phenomenon is often studied via choice-based paradigms. This rapidly advancing field of neuroscience is newly being applied to psychiatry, using neuroimaging and computational approaches.[15]

REWARD SYSTEMS

Reward is a broad construct that can encompass innate rewards like food, as well as learned or complex reinforcers. Among healthy individuals, food and money are commonly used to evaluate reward responsiveness. This pattern creates a complexity in adapting experimental designs, because the reward value of food cannot be assumed in eating disorders. Reward learning can theoretically include both positive and negative feedback, although learning from positive feedback is better understood, to date.

Numerous studies have measured the degree to which individuals with eating disorders find food rewarding, or pleasurable, as compared with healthy controls. Individuals with AN rate food as less pleasurable than healthy controls, especially high-calorie foods.[16] Some have hypothesized that individuals with AN do not experience food as rewarding, and that this experience results in decreased intake.[17–19]

Individuals with BN have high scores on self-report measures of novelty, pleasure, and sensation-seeking behaviors.[20] Moreover, the self-reported drive to eat for pleasure in the absence of an energy deficit predicts the development of loss-of-control eating[21] and is associated with binge eating frequency.[22]

Patients with AN and BN consume large amounts of artificial sweetener through gum, diet beverages, and sweetener packets as compared with healthy controls.[23] Together, these observations have led to the bottom-up examination of reward systems through behavioral and neuroimaging experiments.

Behavioral Studies: Anorexia Nervosa

To assess the reward value of food in AN, some studies measure motivation to pursue food, assessed as speed of responding to food (faster response indicates greater motivation). Patients with AN reported less wanting of high-calorie foods and response times were slower (than healthy controls) when selecting between

2 high-calorie foods.[17,24] In 1 study (but not the other), individuals with AN were faster than healthy controls to select low-calorie foods.[17]

Approach–avoidance paradigms assume that it is easier to approach than to avoid stimuli with motivational value. Two studies suggest less motivation to pursue food by finding reduced approach bias (approach responding minus avoidance responding) to food stimuli in AN.[25,26] Adolescents with AN displayed an approach bias toward low-calorie, but not high-calorie, food stimuli.[27] Individuals with AN, and the binge eating/purging subtype in particular, showed greater motivation than healthy controls to obtain artificial sweetener.[28]

Reward learning is understudied in AN, especially using behavioral tasks. One study has demonstrated that individuals with AN are impaired at learning from feedback, both before and after weight restoration.[29]

Brain Studies: Anorexia Nervosa

Many functional MRI (fMRI) studies have presented images of food (presumed to be innately rewarding) and noted differential activation among AN in areas of the brain that are considered parts of the reward system (ventral striatum, middle frontal gyrus, ventromedial PFC), and dorsolateral PFC (dlPFC), although specific regions and the direction of neural activation differ across studies (eg, hypoactivity vs hyperactivity).[30–33] Some studies have shown differences between AN and healthy controls in response to sweet taste, although in regions less central to reward.[34–36]

In monetary tasks, underweight adolescents with AN appropriately differentiated between wins and losses in the ventral striatum,[37] whereas adults recovered from AN demonstrated hyporesponsiveness to monetary rewards in the ventral striatum compared with healthy controls.[38]

The reward system has also been probed by measuring neural response to the differences between received and expected rewards, the so-called prediction error. In eating disorders, this phenomenon has been studied by training associations between neutral stimuli and delivery of aliquots of sweet liquid (presumed reward). When prediction error occurred, there were differences between patients with AN and healthy controls in neural activation patterns in the striatum, as well as in the OFC.[39,40]

Indications of reward system abnormalities also come from PET studies, which have identified increased dopamine receptor (D2/D3) binding in the ventral striatum among individuals recovered from AN.[41,42] Although these data hint at an abnormality in dopamine pathways, 1 PET study of dopamine receptors found no difference between patients with AN and healthy controls.[43] Diffusion tensor imaging approaches and resting state functional connectivity studies have shown increased connectivity within the reward system, specifically the nucleus accumbens–OFC connectivity.[44]

Summary

Together, behavioral and neuroimaging data suggest decreased reward properties of food, abnormal value and/or processing of reward value of food, and hints of abnormal dopamine functioning. Although intriguing, these findings have not been linked directly to disturbances in eating behavior in AN.

Behavioral Studies: Bulimia Nervosa

To measure the reward value of food among individuals with BN, 2 studies have assessed how hard patients will work for food (ie, motivation). In 1 study, women with BN worked harder than healthy controls for chocolate candies, which were delivered and consumed as they were earned, providing immediate reinforcement.[45] In another, women with BN pressed buttons to earn points to be cashed in at the end of the experiment for aliquots of a palatable yogurt shake. When instructed to binge eat, individuals with BN worked harder for the shake than healthy controls. However, when specifically told to work toward a comfortable level of intake and not to binge eat, individuals with BN did not work as hard as healthy controls for the yogurt shake portions.[46] To measure the reinforcing value of taste without ingestion, 1 study used a modified sham feeding procedure during which participants sipped and spit solutions as much as they wanted in 1-minute increments. Women with BN sipped roughly 50% more than healthy controls, regardless of solution sweetness.[47] These experiments indicate an increased reinforcing value of food and of the orosensory aspects of eating among women with BN. There are currently no experiments with a nonfood reward, leaving a gap in understanding reward processing and reward learning in BN.

Brain Studies: Bulimia Nervosa

Neural responses to pictures of food or actual tastes have been somewhat inconsistent across studies of BN. Participants with BN often show greater activation in the medial OFC, anterior cingulate cortex (ACC), visual cortex, and insula in response to pictures of palatable foods relative to healthy controls,[48,49] and this increased activation has been correlated with symptom severity.[49] Negative mood states before scanning have been associated with increased neural activation in anticipation of a palatable milkshake, suggesting a link between affect and food evaluation.[50]

In contrast, some research suggests a reduced reward response both to expected sweet taste receipt and to unexpected taste receipt in BN relative to healthy controls.[51–53] Women remitted from BN have been found to have increased neural response to predictable receipt of palatable foods and an abnormal failure to devalue taste stimuli after eating.[54,55] In a fed state compared with a fasted state, individuals remitted from BN do not show the decrease in putamen and amygdala responses to liquid tastants (sucrose or water) that healthy controls do.[56]

Unlike healthy controls, individuals remitted from BN did not differentiate between wins and losses in ventral striatum response during a monetary choice task.[57] When visual stimuli were associated with later food and later monetary rewards, individuals with BN (and binge eating disorder) showed altered activation to food-associated stimuli, but no significant group differences related to monetary reward.[58]

In the prediction error paradigm, adults with BN showed decreased activation in the bilateral ventral putamen, amygdala, insula, and lateral OFC associated with unexpected outcomes related to receipt of sucrose and prediction errors.[53] Thus, neural signals involved in reward-based learning may be altered in both adolescent and adult BN.

Structurally, voxel-based morphometry has shown increased[59] or normal[60] volumes of ventral striatum (nucleus accumbens) among individuals with BN compared with healthy controls. PET and single photon emission computed tomography studies have identified decreased striatal dopamine transporter availability and decreased dorsal striatal dopamine release associated with binge eating frequency among individuals with BN.[61,62] Very few published studies have focused on resting state functional connectivity in individuals with BN.[63–66] These studies have focused on somatosensory, dorsal ACC, and cerebellar seeds and networks, not reward circuitry. However, integrations of graph theory network analysis approaches with resting state data suggest that women with BN show reduced nodal strength in reward-related areas (the medial OFC and putamen).[66] Moreover, increases in reward-circuit connectivity (from the ACC to ventral striatum and anterior insula) after repetitive transcranial magnetic stimulation was associated with symptom remission, suggesting that increases in reward circuitry connectivity may mediate symptom improvement.[67]

Summary
Together, behavioral and neuroimaging studies suggest an increased reinforcing value of food and changes in the brain reward system in association with food. There is, as yet, little evidence to suggest non–food-related reward system abnormalities.

BEHAVIORAL AND COGNITIVE CONTROL

The broad constructs of behavioral and cognitive control include motor inhibition and attentional control.[68] Behavioral paradigms that assess behavioral and cognitive control typically require individuals to inhibit a response or ignore interfering information. For example, go/no-go tasks measure action restraint and require the inhibition of a button-pressing go response when no-go stimuli appear on a screen.[69] Stop-signal tasks require withholding of a button-pressing go response when a rare auditory or visual stop signal sounds or appears.[68,70] The delay between the go and the stop signal varies across the task, resulting in easy (short delay) and more difficult (long delay) trials. The Stroop task[71] and Simon task[72] require individuals to override a prepotent response when 2 pieces of information are inconsistent (eg, naming a word's ink color instead of reading the color word such as blue, pressing a button that matches the direction in which an arrow is pointing rather than the side of the screen on which it is presented). Overlapping corticostriatothalamocortical loops, including lateral PFC, ACC, dorsal striatum, the presupplementary motor area, insula, and parietal regions, are involved in these processes.[73,74]

Behavioral control deficits may be particularly relevant to the pathophysiology of binge eating, because the sense of loss of control over eating is a defining element of binge episodes in the binge eating/purging subtype of AN and in BN.[75] In AN, recent theories posit that increased cognitive control and difficulties with set shifting may promote or maintain excessive control over food intake.[76] In addition to difficulty controlling eating, high rates of other dysregulated, often impulsive behaviors among individuals with BN suggest that the disorder may also be characterized by impairment in inhibitory control across multiple domains.[77–81]

Behavioral Studies: Anorexia Nervosa

Neuropsychological studies of individuals with AN have consistently found executive function deficits in some domains related to cognitive control. Patients with AN show difficulty changing responses when instructions changed, as evidenced on set shifting tasks and Stroop tasks.[82] Although attention is often impaired owing to starvation, studies of attention bias do not suggest deficits in attentional control among individuals with AN.[83] Behavioral control tasks, in which participants must engage inhibitory control to prevent an active motor response, generally do not show a difference between individuals with AN and healthy controls.[84]

Brain Studies: Anorexia Nervosa

Despite the numerous reports of cognitive inflexibility in AN, the neural correlates are not clear. One study that required shifting of behavioral responses found less activation in the frontostriatal circuits and associated increased set shifting errors among individuals with AN.[85] Several studies found decreased neural activation in regions that are considered part of control networks during tasks that involve inhibition of motor responses. On the stop signal task, there are data suggesting decreased medial prefrontal activity during difficult trials; however, there is no evidence of behavioral differences between patients with AN and healthy controls.[84,86,87]

Summary
Behavior in AN is highly suggestive of aberrant self-control processes; neuroimaging suggests that the neural mechanisms of AN symptoms may be more complex than solely excessive self-control.

Behavioral Studies: Bulimia Nervosa

Behavioral data from classic neurocognitive paradigms support the hypothesis that BN is characterized by deficits in both behavioral and cognitive control. Results of a metaanalysis that included mostly studies using Stroop task variants suggest deficits in cognitive control, or interference control, in individuals with BN that are more pronounced when food or body-related stimuli are used.[88]

Brain Studies: Bulimia Nervosa

In food-related fMRI studies, individuals with BN show altered neural activation in control-related regions. Individuals with BN showed decreased activation compared with healthy controls in the left dlPFC in response to food pictures and trend-level decreased left dlPFC activation during chocolate shake receipt.[49,52] However, because there is no explicit control-related demand during these tasks, decreased activation in PFC cannot be linked explicitly to control-related processes.

To date, 4 studies have used cognitive and behavioral tasks during fMRI scanning to measure the neural correlates of control in BN. Two studies found that both adolescents and adults with BN showed decreased activation in the frontostriatal control circuitry during the resolution of cognitive conflict on the Simon task, and this decreased activation was associated with more frequent bulimic symptoms.[89,90] Machine learning approaches using these altered patterns of activation can reliably distinguish BN cases from healthy controls.[91,92] One study has used a go/no-go task to examine differences in response inhibition to food and neutral images and found that only a BN subgroup with the most frequent binge eating showed decreased activation during response inhibition to neutral images in dorsal striatum, with additional hypoactivation in sensorimotor areas.[92] One emotional go/no-go study found that individuals with BN showed age-dependent deficits in PFC activation during emotional go/no-go task response inhibition relative to healthy controls.[93]

Structural neuroimaging findings also suggest that alterations in control-related circuitry in BN may be age dependent and reflect an abnormal neurodevelopmental trajectory. Cross-sectional data from large samples of adolescents and adults with BN indicate age-associated decreases in the volume and cortical thickness of frontal and parietal regions.[94,95] The only longitudinal structural imaging study of adolescent BN to date reported that reduced cortical thickness compared with healthy controls in the right ventrolateral PFC persisted over 2 years of follow-up, even among those who achieved symptom remission.[96] Between-subject variations in cortical thickness of the ventrolateral PFC were inversely associated with specific BN symptoms, suggesting consistently more pronounced cortical thinning in this control-associated region in individuals with more frequent BN symptoms. Subcortical findings have been more inconsistent, and decreased[60,97] or normal[98,99] volumes of dorsal striatum, specifically the caudate nucleus, have been documented in BN compared with control participants.

The only published study of brain connectivity at rest using a control-related seed (in the left dlPFC) did not report any difference in resting state functional connectivity in executive control circuitry in women with BN compared with healthy controls.[63]

Summary
Behavioral data in BN indicate deficits in inhibitory control that are particularly pronounced in the context of food cues. Limited existing neuroimaging data suggest that functional and structural alterations in control circuits occur early in the course of BN and may contribute to the disorder's persistence over time.

DECISION MAKING

Several important advances in cognitive neuroscience have come from examining decision making. Examining maladaptive behavior in eating disorders creates top-down models and testable hypotheses about neural mechanisms of illness. This approach has been less commonly used to date, but holds a lot of promise. Decision making is often measured as a choice behavior, which in many ways is the result of reward and control as well as other cognitive processes such as attention, learning, and memory. This approach, which integrates behavioral and brain studies, provides complementary insights to the bottom-up probes described elsewhere in this article.

Activation in corticostriatal regions (caudate, anterior putamen, ventromedial PFC, and dlPFC) is integral to goal-directed action.[4,100–104] Computational approaches have allowed for differentiation between goal-oriented and more automatic decisions.[105] Value-based decision making has been shown to be mediated by cortical systems.[106,107] When decisions are more automatic, or habitual, these processes are related to the dorsal striatum and associated cortical regions.[108]

Monetary Decisions (Temporal Discounting)

One well-characterized behavior involves the trade-off between rewards available immediately, and rewards available only after a delay—termed temporal discounting. Among healthy controls, there is individual variability in the rate at which the value of the reward decreases with the time needed to wait to receive it. This complex behavior incorporates reward systems and control systems, as well as the experience of time.[109] The discount rate, a quantification of the loss of value over time, has been shown to relate to real-life behaviors, such as academic performance and risk-taking behaviors. Among individuals with eating disorders, temporal discounting has been of interest because of the potential analogy to trade-offs between the immediate food reward and longer term weight- or shape-related goals.[110] Several studies have found that individuals with AN discount the value of money less steeply than healthy controls,[111–114] although some have not.[115,116] Associated neuroimaging findings have suggested that there are frontostriatal system differences between patients with AN and healthy controls during temporal discounting. Acutely ill individuals with AN showed decreased ventral striatal and dorsal ACC activation associated with decreased (ie, less steep) discounting of money. After weight restoration, normalization of behavior was associated with increased activation of the striatum and dlPFC (as well as other cortical regions).[112] In a different paradigm, while healthy controls showed different activation patterns in reward and cognitive control-related circuitry depending on metabolic state (ie, hunger vs satiety), individuals recovered from AN did not.[117]

Among individuals with BN, temporal discounting rates are greater than those of healthy controls, suggesting a preference for immediate reward, difficulty delaying gratification, and perhaps poor control over reward.[118,119] Transcranial direct current stimulation over the dlPFC decreased temporal discounting rates and temporarily decreased urges to binge eat.[120] Although no published fMRI studies of BN have used delay discounting tasks, these noninvasive brain stimulation data support the hypothesis that lateral PFC dysfunction in BN contributes to difficulty delaying gratification.

Food-Based Decisions

Disturbances in eating are the central behavioral phenomena defining eating disorders (see **Fig. 1**). Examining the neural mechanisms of these maladaptive behaviors are therefore the main focus of a top-down approach. To address this in AN, a food choice task asks participants to make choices about what to eat, knowing that they will receive one of their choices after the task.[106,121] Choice of high-fat foods during the task has been shown to correlate with actual caloric intake in a laboratory meal, providing external validation that this task measures maladaptive restrictive intake.[122] One proposed model suggests that these maladaptive behaviors are habitual, or over-trained, choices and not governed by value-based decision-making systems.[123] A key prediction of this model is that, like neural mechanisms of habit, restricted food intake in AN is guided by activity in the dorsal striatum and associated cortical regions, such as the dlPFC. fMRI scanning during this food choice task indicated that among those with AN, but not healthy controls, active food choice was associated with neural activation in the dorsal striatum.

SUMMARY

Research on the neural mechanisms of AN and BN have yet to converge on 1 clear underlying pathophysiology. Yet, current directions in research are promising. The most compelling data come from studies that began with a biological model and tested specific hypotheses. These behavioral, functional, and structural MRI, and PET studies have indicated that the reinforcing value of food is reduced in AN, whereas individuals with BN experience greater reinforcement from properties of food that are associated with binge eating. There are hints of reward processing and reward learning abnormalities that indicate that reward system dysfunction may be an important path forward. Current data suggest that control systems—broadly focused on corticostriatothalamocortical pathways—are affected in BN, and may reflect altered neurodevelopment. This direction has been less fruitful for understanding AN. Direct examination of maladaptive behavior in AN has indicated that there are differences in neural mechanisms of decision making about food. By testing hypotheses about the neural mechanisms of maladaptive behavior and about illness-related dysfunction in reward and control systems, the field may advance in understanding the pathophysiology of eating disorders.

Considerations and Limitations of Existing Research

Neurocognitive and neuroimaging research in AN and BN have often been limited by small sample sizes and differences in task designs that impact interpretation. For example, probes of the reinforcing value of food tend to find decreased reward from food in AN. Yet, when an active response to a reward or an actual ingestion is the outcome, there is less evidence of decreased responding (or sensitivity) to reward. Predictability of the stimulus delivered, the reward stimulus used (eg, pictures of money or food; glucose, sucrose, or sweet–fat combination solutions; artificial saliva; noncaloric sweet taste), and responses measured (eg, passive receipt, approach or avoidance responses) contribute to challenges in clarifying dysfunction in reward systems.

Studies of control mechanisms have used complex tasks with multiple subcomponents. For example, because the Stroop and Simon tasks simultaneously assess inhibitory and attentional control and conflict monitoring, it is unclear whether high error rates on these tasks indicate deficits in one or all of these dimensions of control, making it difficult to clarify mechanism dysfunction in eating disorders.

Probing decision making around monetary choices has its limitations, because this is not a direct reflection of the pathology of eating disorders. It may be that probing discounting in the setting of more illness-specific choices will be fruitful.[124]

There are also universal challenges in interpreting neural correlates in the setting of illness. If a clinical group performs differently from healthy controls on a task, differences in brain activation may simply reflect that behavior—without relevance for disease processes. When groups perform similarly on a task, several factors (eg, a different cognitive process, a different neural computation) could explain reduced activation in a clinical group, and again relevance to disease processes cannot be assumed automatically.[125] Throughout the literature, differences in the stage of illness of the studied population creates a challenge. The field would benefit from clearer definitions of clinical stages, to improve our ability to identify markers of disease.

Future Directions

To move the field forward, new tasks, analytical approaches, and longitudinal designs are needed. Novel paradigms that permit a top-down approach may better elucidate the neural mechanisms of illness. Many existing paradigms have not demonstrated relevance to actual maladaptive behavior. Several studies report statistical correlations between eating disorder symptoms and control-related measures, yet it is unknown whether the processes assessed by these tasks directly promote salient pathology in AN and BN. Tasks that measure eating-specific planning[126] and decision making, and food approach followed by consumption will be important to more accurately model the neural bases of dysregulated eating in AN and BN.

Tasks with greater specificity around subcomponents of broad neurocognitive constructs could help to inform future top-down studies and isolate targets for novel intervention. For example, within the realm of cognitive control, some data suggest that investigation of attentional control in eating disorders is warranted.[79,94,127,128] This process may contribute to difficulty in planning and organizing eating behavior in BN.[127]

Advanced analytical approaches such as computational models show a lot of promise for understanding circuit-level abnormalities and individual variability that may promote eating disorder symptoms. Models from other areas of computational psychiatry could be developed to specifically understand reward, control, and decision-making processes in food and non–food-based paradigms.

All of these directions need to be incorporated into longitudinal imaging studies with large samples to fully understand the neuropathology of eating disorders.

REFERENCES

1. Kaye W. Neurobiology of anorexia and bulimia nervosa. Physiol Behav 2008; 94(1):121–35.
2. Kaye WH, Wierenga CE, Bailer UF, et al. Nothing tastes as good as skinny feels: the neurobiology of anorexia nervosa. Trends Neurosci 2013;36(2):110–20.
3. Berridge KC, Robinson TE, Aldridge JW. Dissecting components of reward: 'liking', 'wanting', and learning. Curr Opin Pharmacol 2009;9(1):65–73.
4. Balleine BW, Dickinson A. Goal-directed instrumental action: contingency and incentive learning and their cortical substrates. Neuropharmacology 1998;37: 407–19.

5. Keating C, Tilbrook AJ, Rossell SL, et al. Reward processing in anorexia nervosa. Neuropsychologia 2012;50(5):567–75.
6. Pearson CM, Wonderlich SA, Smith GT. A risk and maintenance model for bulimia nervosa: from impulsive action to compulsive behavior. Psychol Rev 2015;122(3):516–35.
7. Chambers CD, Garavan H, Bellgrove MA. Insights into the neural basis of response inhibition from cognitive and clinical neuroscience. Neurosci Biobehav Rev 2009;33(5):631–46.
8. Aron AR. From reactive to proactive and selective control: developing a richer model for stopping inappropriate responses. Biol Psychiatry 2011;69(12): e55–68.
9. Dosenbach NU, Fair DA, Miezin FM, et al. Distinct brain networks for adaptive and stable task control in humans. Proc Natl Acad Sci U S A 2007;104(26): 11073–8.
10. Haber SN. Corticostriatal circuitry. In: Pfaff DW, Volkow ND, editors. Neuroscience in the 21st century. New York: Springer New York; 2016. p. 1–21.
11. Hampshire A, Chamberlain SR, Monti MM, et al. The role of the right inferior frontal gyrus: inhibition and attentional control. Neuroimage 2010;50:1313–9.
12. Miller EK, Cohen JD. An integrative theory of prefrontal cortex function. Annu Rev Neurosci 2001;24:167–202.
13. Fischer S, Smith GT, Cyders MA. Another look at impulsivity: a meta-analytic review comparing specific dispositions to rash action in their relationship to bulimic symptoms. Clin Psychol Rev 2008;28(8):1413–25.
14. Marsh R, Maia TV, Peterson BS. Functional disturbances within frontostriatal circuits across multiple childhood psychopathologies. Am J Psychiatry 2009; 166(6):664–74.
15. Maia TV, Frank MJ. From reinforcement learning models to psychiatric and neurological disorders. Nat Neurosci 2011;14(2):154–62.
16. Lloyd CE, Steinglass JE. What can food-image tasks teach us about anorexia nervosa? A systematic review. J Eat Disord 2018;6(31):1–18.
17. Cowdrey FA, Finlayson G, Park RJ. Liking compared with wanting for high- and low-calorie foods in anorexia nervosa: aberrant food reward even after weight restoration. Am J Clin Nutr 2013;97(3):463–70.
18. Berridge KC. 'Liking' and 'wanting' food rewards: brain substrates and roles in eating disorders. Physiol Behav 2009;97(5):537–50.
19. Davis C, Woodside DB. Sensitivity to the rewarding effects of food and exercise in the eating disorders. Compr Psychiatry 2002;43(3):189–94.
20. Wagner A, Barbarich N, Frank G, et al. Personality traits after recovery from eating disorders: do subtypes differ? Int J Eat Disord 2006;39(4):276–84.
21. Lowe MR, Arigo D, Butryn ML, et al. Hedonic hunger prospectively predicts onset and maintenance of loss of control eating among college women. Health Psychol 2016;35(3):238.
22. Witt AA, Lowe MR. Hedonic hunger and binge eating among women with eating disorders. Int J Eat Disord 2014;47(3):273–80.
23. Klein DA, Boudreau GS, Devlin MJ, et al. Artificial sweetener use among individuals with eating disorders. Int J Eat Disord 2006;39(4):341–5.
24. Scaife JC, Godier LR, Reinecke A, et al. Differential activation of the frontal pole to high vs low calorie foods: the neural basis of food preference in anorexia nervosa? Psychiatry Res 2016;258:44–53.
25. Veenstra EM, de Jong PJ. Reduced automatic motivational orientation towards food in restricting anorexia nervosa. J Abnorm Psychol 2011;120(3):708–18.

26. Paslakis G, Kühn S, Schaubschläger A, et al. Explicit and implicit approach vs. avoidance tendencies towards high vs. low calorie food cues in patients with anorexia nervosa and healthy controls. Appetite 2016;107:171–9.

27. Neimeijer RA, de Jong PJ, Roefs A. Automatic approach/avoidance tendencies towards food and the course of anorexia nervosa. Appetite 2015;91:28–34.

28. Schebendach J, Klein DA, Mayer LES, et al. Assessment of the motivation to use artificial sweetener among individuals with an eating disorder. Appetite 2017; 109:131–6.

29. Foerde K, Steinglass JE. Decreased feedback learning in anorexia nervosa persists after weight restoration. Int J Eat Disord 2017;50(4):415–23.

30. Fuglset TS, Landro NI, Reas DL, et al. Functional brain alterations in anorexia nervosa: a scoping review. J Eat Disord 2016;4:32.

31. Cowdrey FA, Park RJ, Harmer CJ, et al. Increased neural processing of rewarding and aversive food stimuli in recovered anorexia nervosa. Biol Psychiatry 2011;70(8):736–43.

32. Ellison Z, Foong J, Howard R, et al. Functional anatomy of calorie fear in anorexia nervosa. Lancet 1998;352:1192.

33. Holsen LM, Lawson EA, Blum J, et al. Food motivation circuitry hypoactivation related to hedonic and nonhedonic aspects of hunger and satiety in women with active anorexia nervosa and weight-restored women with anorexia nervosa. J Psychiatry Neurosci 2012;37(5):322–32.

34. Oberndorfer TA, Frank GK, Simmons AN, et al. Altered insula response to sweet taste processing after recovery from anorexia and bulimia nervosa. Am J Psychiatry 2013;170(10):1143–51.

35. Wagner A, Aizenstein H, Mazurkewicz L, et al. Altered insula response to taste stimuli in individuals recovered from restricting-type anorexia nervosa. Neuropsychopharmacology 2008;33(3):513–23.

36. Monteleone AM, Monteleone P, Esposito F, et al. Altered processing of rewarding and aversive basic taste stimuli in symptomatic women with anorexia nervosa and bulimia nervosa: an fMRI study. J Psychiatr Res 2017;90:94–101.

37. Bischoff-Grethe A, McCurdy D, Grenesko-Stevens E, et al. Altered brain response to reward and punishment in adolescents with anorexia nervosa. Psychiatry Res 2013;214(3):331–40.

38. Wagner A, Aizenstein H, Venkatraman VK, et al. Altered reward processing in women recovered from anorexia nervosa. Am J Psychiatry 2007;164(12): 1842–9.

39. Frank GK, Reynolds JR, Shott ME, et al. Anorexia nervosa and obesity are associated with opposite brain reward response. Neuropsychopharmacology 2012; 37(9):2031–46.

40. Frank GKW, DeGuzman MC, Shott ME, et al. Association of brain reward learning response with harm avoidance, weight gain, and hypothalamic effective connectivity in adolescent anorexia nervosa. JAMA Psychiatry 2018; 75(10):1071–80.

41. Frank GK, Bailer UF, Henry SE, et al. Increased dopamine D2/D3 receptor binding after recovery from anorexia nervosa measured by positron emission tomography and [11c]raclopride. Biol Psychiatry 2005;58(11):908–12.

42. Bailer UF, Frank GK, Henry SE, et al. Serotonin transporter binding after recovery from eating disorders. Psychopharmacology (Berl) 2007;195(3):315–24.

43. Broft A, Slifstein M, Osborne J, et al. Striatal dopamine type 2 receptor availability in anorexia nervosa. Psychiatry Res 2015;233(3):380–7.

44. Cha J, Ide JS, Bowman FD, et al. Abnormal reward circuitry in anorexia nervosa: a longitudinal, multimodal MRI study. Hum Brain Mapp 2016;37(11):3835–46.
45. Bodell L, Keel P. Weight suppression in bulimia nervosa: associations with biology and behavior. J Abnorm Psychol 2015;124(4):994–1002.
46. Schebendach J, Broft A, Foltin R, et al. Can the reinforcing value of food be measured in bulimia nervosa? Appetite 2013;62:70–5.
47. Klein D, Schenbendach J, Brown A, et al. Modified sham feeding of sweet solutions in women with and without bulimia nervosa. Physiol Behav 2009;96(1):44–50.
48. Brooks S, O'Daly O, Uher R, et al. Differential neural responses to food images in women with bulimia versus anorexia nervosa. PLoS One 2011;6(7):1–8.
49. Uher R, Murphy T, Brammer M, et al. Medial prefrontal cortex activity associated with symptom provocation in eating disorders. Am J Psychiatry 2004;161(7):1238–46.
50. Bohon C, Stice E. Negative affect and neural response to palatable food intake in bulimia nervosa. Appetite 2012;58(3):964–70.
51. Frank G, Wagner A, Brooks-Achenbach S, et al. Altered brain activity in women recovered from bulimic type eating disorders after a glucose challenge. A pilot study. Int J Eat Disord 2006;39(1):76–9.
52. Bohon C, Stice E. Reward abnormalities among women with full and subthreshold bulimia nervosa: a functional magnetic resonance imaging study. Int J Eat Disord 2011;44(7):585–95.
53. Frank G, Reynolds J, Shott M, et al. Altered temporal difference learning in bulimia nervosa. Biol Psychiatry 2011;70(8):728–35.
54. Oberndorfer T, Frank G, Fudge J, et al. Altered insula response to sweet taste processing after recovery from anorexia and bulimia nervosa. Am J Psychiatry 2013;214(2):132–41.
55. Radeloff D, Willmann K, Otto L, et al. High-fat taste challenge reveals altered striatal response in women recovered from bulimia nervosa: a pilot study. World J Biol Psychiatry 2014;15(4):307–16.
56. Ely A, Wierenga C, Bischoff-Grethe A, et al. Response in taste circuitry is not modulated by hunger and satiety in women remitted from bulimia nervosa. J Abnorm Psychol 2017;126(5):519–30.
57. Wagner A, Aizeinstein H, Venkatraman V, et al. Altered striatal response to reward in bulimia nervosa after recovery. Int J Eat Disord 2010;43(4):289–94.
58. Simon J, Skunde M, Walther S, et al. Neural signature of food reward processing in bulimic-type eating disorders. Soc Cogn Affect Neurosci 2016;11(9):1393–401.
59. Schafer A, Vaitl D, Schienle A. Regional grey matter volume abnormalities in bulimia nervosa and binge-eating disorder. Neuroimage 2010;50(2):639–43.
60. Frank GK, Shott ME, Hagman JO, et al. Alterations in brain structures related to taste reward circuitry in ill and recovered anorexia nervosa and in bulimia nervosa. Am J Psychiatry 2013;170(10):1152–60.
61. Broft A, Shingleton R, Kaufman J, et al. Striatal dopamine in bulimia nervosa: a PET imaging study. Int J Eat Disord 2012;45(5):648–56.
62. Tauscher J, Pirker W, Willeit M, et al. [123I] beta-CIT and single photon emission computed tomography reveal reduced brain serotonin transporter availability in bulimia nervosa. Biol Psychiatry 2001;49(4):326–32.
63. Lavagnino L, Amianto F, D'Agata F, et al. Reduced resting-state functional connectivity of the somatosensory cortex predicts psychopathological symptoms in women with bulimia nervosa. Front Behav Neurosci 2014;8:270.

64. Lee S, Ran Kim K, Ku J, et al. Resting-state synchrony between anterior cingulate cortex and precuneus relates to body shape concern in anorexia nervosa and bulimia nervosa. Psychiatry Res 2014;221(1):43–8.
65. Amianto F, D'Agata F, Lavagnino L, et al. Intrinsic connectivity networks within cerebellum and beyond in eating disorders. Cerebellum 2013;12(5):623–31.
66. Wang L, Kong Q-M, Li K, et al. Altered intrinsic functional brain architecture in female patients with bulimia nervosa. J Psychiatry Neurosci 2017;42(6):414–23.
67. Dunlop K, Woodside B, Lam E, et al. Increases in frontostriatal connectivity are associated with response to dorsomedial repetitive transcranial magnetic stimulation in refractory binge/purge behaviors. Neuroimage Clin 2015;8:611–8.
68. Eagle D, Bari A, Robbins T. The neuropsychopharmacology of action inhibition: cross-species translation of the stop-signal and go/no-go tasks. Psychopharmacology 2008;199:439–56.
69. Rubia K, Russelol T, Overmeyer S, et al. Mapping motor inhibition: conjunctive brain activations across different versions of go/no-go and stop tasks. Neuroimage 2001;13(2):250–61.
70. Logan G, Schachar R, Tannock R. Impulsivity and inhibitory control. Psychol Sci 1997;8:60–4.
71. Stroop J. Studies of interference in serial verbal reactions. J Exp Psychol 1935; 18:643–62.
72. Simon JR. Reactions toward the source of stimulation. J Exp Psychol 1969; 81(1):174–6.
73. Aron AR, Herz DM, Brown P, et al. Frontosubthalamic circuits for control of action and cognition. J Neurosci 2016;36(45):11489–95.
74. Petersen SE, Posner MI. The attention system of the human brain: 20 years after. Annu Rev Neurosci 2012;35:73–89.
75. American Psychiatric Association. Diagnostic and statistical manual of mental disorders: fifth edition (DSM-5). Washington, DC: American Psychiatric Association; 2013.
76. Wierenga C, Ely A, Bischoff-Grethe A, et al. Are extremes of consumption in eating disorders related to an altered balance between reward and inhibition? Front Behav Neurosci 2014;9(8):410.
77. Fischer S, Smith GT, Anderson KG. Clarifying the role of impulsivity in bulimia nervosa. Int J Eat Disord 2003;33:406–11.
78. Nasser J, Gluck M, Geliebter A. Impulsivity and test meal intake in obese binge eating women. Appetite 2004;43(3):303–7.
79. Rosval L, Steiger H, Bruce K, et al. Impulsivity in women with eating disorders: problem of response inhibition, planning, or attention? Int J Eat Disord 2006; 39(7):590–3.
80. Steiger H, Lehoux P, Gauvin L. Impulsivity, dietary control and the urge to binge in bulimic syndromes. Int J Eat Disord 1999;26(3):261–74.
81. Yanovski S, Nelson J, Dubbert B, et al. Association of binge eating disorder and psychiatric comorbidity in obese subjects. Am J Psychiatry 1993;150(10): 1472–9.
82. Smith KE, Mason TB, Johnson JS, et al. A systematic review of reviews of neurocognitive functioning in eating disorders: the state-of-the-literature and future directions. Int J Eat Disord 2018. [Epub ahead of print].
83. Schneier FR, Kimeldorf MB, Choo TH, et al. Attention bias in adults with anorexia nervosa, obsessive-compulsive disorder, and social anxiety disorder. J Psychiatr Res 2016;79:61–9.

84. Bartholdy S, Dalton B, O'Daly OG, et al. A systematic review of the relationship between eating, weight and inhibitory control using the stop signal task. Neurosci Biobehav Rev 2016;64:35–62.

85. Zastrow A, Kaiser S, Stippich C, et al. Neural correlates of impaired cognitive-behavioral flexibility in anorexia nervosa. Am J Psychiatry 2009;166(5):608–16.

86. Wierenga C, Bischoff-Grethe A, Melrose AJ, et al. Altered BOLD response during inhibitory and error processing in adolescents with anorexia nervosa. PLoS One 2014;9(3):e92017.

87. Oberndorfer TA, Kaye WH, Simmons AN, et al. Demand-specific alteration of medial prefrontal cortex response during an inhibition task in recovered anorexic women. Int J Eat Disord 2011;44(1):1–8.

88. Wu M, Hartmann M, Skunde M, et al. Inhibitory control in bulimic-type eating disorders: a systematic review and meta-analysis. PLoS One 2013;8(12):e83412.

89. Marsh R, Steinglass JE, Gerber AJ, et al. Deficient activity in the neural systems that mediate self-regulatory control in bulimia nervosa. Arch Gen Psychiatry 2009;66(1):51–63.

90. Marsh R, Horga G, Wang Z, et al. An FMRI study of self-regulatory control and conflict resolution in adolescents with bulimia nervosa. Am J Psychiatry 2011; 168(11):1210–20.

91. Cyr M, Yang X, Horga G, et al. Abnormal fronto-striatal activation as a marker of threshold and subthreshold bulimia nervosa. Hum Brain Mapp 2018;39(4): 1796–804.

92. Skunde M, Walther S, Simon JJ, et al. Neural signature of behavioural inhibition in women with bulimia nervosa. J Psychiatry Neurosci 2016;41(5):E69–78.

93. Dreyfuss MFW, Riegel ML, Pedersen GA, et al. Patients with bulimia nervosa do not show typical neurodevelopment of cognitive control under emotional influences. Psychiatry Res Neuroimaging 2017;266:59–65.

94. Berner LA, Stefan M, Lee S, et al. Altered cortical thickness and attentional deficits in adolescent girls and women with bulimia nervosa. J Psychiatry Neurosci 2018;43(3):151–60.

95. Marsh R, Stefan M, Bansal R, et al. Anatomical characteristics of the cerebral surface in bulimia nervosa. Biol Psychiatry 2015;77(7):616–23.

96. Cyr M, Kopala-Sibley DC, Lee S, et al. Reduced inferior and orbital frontal thickness in adolescent bulimia nervosa persists over two-year follow-up. J Am Acad Child Adolesc Psychiatry 2017;56(10):866–74.e7.

97. Coutinho J, Ramos AF, Maia L, et al. Volumetric alterations in the nucleus accumbens and caudate nucleus in bulimia nervosa: a structural magnetic resonance imaging study. Int J Eat Disord 2015;48(2):206–14.

98. Joos A, Kloppel S, Hartmann A, et al. Voxel-based morphometry in eating disorders: correlation of psychopathology with grey matter volume. Psychiatry Res 2010;182(2):146–51.

99. Amianto F, Caroppo P, D'Agata F, et al. Brain volumetric abnormalities in patients with anorexia and bulimia nervosa: a voxel-based morphometry study. Psychiatry Res 2013;213(3):210–6.

100. de Wit S, Corlett PR, Aitken MR, et al. Differential engagement of the ventromedial prefrontal cortex by goal-directed and habitual behavior toward food pictures in humans. J Neurosci 2009;29(36):11330–8.

101. de Wit S, Watson P, Harsay HA, et al. Corticostriatal connectivity underlies individual differences in the balance between habitual and goal-directed action control. J Neurosci 2012;32(35):12066–75.

102. Balleine BW, O'Doherty JP. Human and rodent homologies in action control: corticostriatal determinants of goal-directed and habitual action. Neuropsychopharmacology 2009;35(1):48–69.

103. Valentin VV, Dickinson A, O'Doherty JP. Determining the neural substrates of goal-directed learning in the human brain. J Neurosci 2007;27(15):4019–26.

104. Tanaka SC, Balleine BW, O'Doherty JP. Calculating consequences: brain systems that encode the causal effects of actions. J Neurosci 2008;28(26):6750–5.

105. Doll BB, Shohamy D, Daw ND. Multiple memory systems as substrates for multiple decision systems. Neurobiol Learn Mem 2015;117:4–13.

106. Hare TA, Camerer CF, Rangel A. Self-control in decision-making involves modulation of the vmPFC valuation system. Science 2009;324(5927):646–8.

107. Pisauro MA, Fouragnan E, Retzler C, et al. Neural correlates of evidence accumulation during value-based decisions revealed via simultaneous EEG-fMRI. Nat Commun 2017;8:15808.

108. Smith KS, Graybiel AM. Habit formation coincides with shifts in reinforcement representations in the sensorimotor striatum. J Neurophysiol 2016;115(3): 1487–98.

109. Lempert KM, Steinglass JE, Pinto A, et al. Can delay discounting deliver on the promise of RDoC? Psychol Med 2018;1–10 [Epub ahead of print].

110. McClelland J, Dalton B, Kekic M, et al. A systematic review of temporal discounting in eating disorders and obesity: behavioural and neuroimaging findings. Neurosci Biobehav Rev 2016;71:506–28.

111. Steinglass JE, Lempert KM, Choo TH, et al. Temporal discounting across three psychiatric disorders: anorexia nervosa, obsessive compulsive disorder, and social anxiety disorder. Depress Anxiety 2017;34(5):463–70.

112. Decker JH, Figner B, Steinglass JE. On weight and waiting: delay discounting in anorexia nervosa pretreatment and posttreatment. Biol Psychiatry 2015;78(9): 606–14.

113. Steinglass JE, Figner B, Berkowitz S, et al. Increased capacity to delay reward in anorexia nervosa. J Int Neuropsychol Soc 2012;18(4):773–80.

114. Steward T, Mestre-Bach G, Vintro-Alcaraz C, et al. Delay discounting of reward and impulsivity in eating disorders: from anorexia nervosa to binge eating disorder. Eur Eat Disord Rev 2017;25(6):601–6.

115. King JA, Geisler D, Bernardoni F, et al. Altered neural efficiency of decision making during temporal reward discounting in anorexia nervosa. J Am Acad Child Adolesc Psychiatry 2016;55(11):972–9.

116. Ritschel F, King JA, Geisler D, et al. Temporal delay discounting in acutely ill and weight-recovered patients with anorexia nervosa. Psychol Med 2015;45(6): 1229–39.

117. Wierenga CE, Bischoff-Grethe A, Melrose AJ, et al. Hunger does not motivate reward in women remitted from anorexia nervosa. Biol Psychiatry 2015;77(7): 642–52.

118. Bari A, Robbins TW. Inhibition and impulsivity: behavioral and neural basis of response control. Prog Neurobiol 2013;108:44–79.

119. Kekic M, Bartholdy S, Cheng J, et al. Increased temporal discounting in bulimia nervosa. Int J Eat Disord 2016;49(12):1077–81.

120. Kekic M, McClelland J, Bartholdy S, et al. Single-session transcranial direct current stimulation temporarily improves symptoms, mood, and self-regulatory control in bulimia nervosa: a randomised controlled trial. PLoS One 2017;12(1): e0167606.

121. Steinglass J, Foerde K, Kostro K, et al. Restrictive food intake as a choice–a paradigm for study. Int J Eat Disord 2015;48(1):59–66.
122. Foerde K, Steinglass JE, Shohamy D, et al. Neural mechanisms supporting maladaptive food choices in anorexia nervosa. Nat Neurosci 2015;18(11):1571–3.
123. Walsh BT. The enigmatic persistence of anorexia nervosa. Am J Psychiatry 2013;170(5):477–84.
124. Schreyer CC, Berry MS, Hansen JL, et al. Delay discounting in patients with anorexia nervosa: examining caloric restriction as a reward. International Conference on Eating Disorders. Chicago, IL, April 21, 2018.
125. Poldrack RA. Is "efficiency" a useful concept in cognitive neuroscience? Dev Cogn Neurosci 2015;11:12–7.
126. Pearson CM, Chester DS, Powell D, et al. Investigating the reinforcing value of binge anticipation. Int J Eat Disord 2016;49(6):539–41.
127. Seitz J, Kahraman-Lanzerath B, Legenbauer T, et al. The role of impulsivity, inattention and comorbid ADHD in patients with bulimia nervosa. PLoS One 2013; 8(5):e63891.
128. Strauss E, Sherman EMS, Spreen O. A compendium of neuropsychological tests: administration, norms, and commentary. 3rd edition. New York: Oxford University Press; 2006.

The Microbiome and Eating Disorders

Jochen Seitz, MD[a], Stefanie Trinh, MSc[b], Beate Herpertz-Dahlmann, MD[a],*

KEYWORDS

- Microbiome • Anorexia nervosa • Inflammation • Gut permeability • Autoantibodies
- Gut-brain interaction • Psychobiotics • Nutrition

KEY POINTS

- The human gut microbiome is involved in host metabolism and weight regulation, host protection and immune system development, and gut-brain interaction.
- Patients with anorexia nervosa (AN) show notable changes in their microbiome, for example, reduced diversity and taxa abundance.
- AN-related changes in microbiome could increase gut permeability, inflammation, and autoantibody formation.
- Reduced microbiome diversity in AN may be associated with depressive, anxious, and eating disorder symptoms.
- Microbiome-directed therapies, for example, using nutritional interventions or psychobiotics, could offer additional treatment strategies.

INTRODUCTION

The human body carries at least as many gut microbial cells as total eukaryotic cells.[1] Out of approximately 1000 different gut microbial species, each human being hosts his or her own personal combination of approximately 500 species[2] acting like an individual's "gut microbial fingerprint." The combination of the genetic information of all gut microbes is termed the "gut microbiome" and contains 150 times more genes than the human genome. This colony of gut microbes continuously interacts with the nutritional supply and with the cells of the gut wall and beyond. It helps digest and break down food, furnishing the human body with many essential nutrients that would otherwise not be available—leading to a symbiotic relationship. Gut microbes affect the

Disclosure Statement: The authors state no conflict of interest.
[a] Department of Child and Adolescent Psychiatry, Psychotherapy and Psychosomatics, University Hospital, RWTH University Aachen, Neuenhofer Weg 21, Aachen D-52074, Germany; [b] Institute for Neuroanatomy, University Hospital, RWTH University Aachen, Wendlingweg 2, Aachen D-52074, Germany
* Corresponding author.
E-mail address: jseitz@ukaachen.de

host metabolism and, moreover, hormonal status. They also play an important role in the education of our immune system from the day we are born and thus help regulate inflammatory processes.[3] Not surprisingly, the microbiome seems to play an important role in diseases such as diabetes, inflammatory bowel disease, and arthritis as well as in obesity. Recently, interactions between the gut microbiome and the brain and behavior (ie, the "gut-brain axis") have become the focus of attention. Current research points to causal roles of the microbiome in diseases such as anxiety disorder and depression and in stress-coping mechanisms.[4] These findings are of increasing interest for anorexia nervosa (AN), where metabolic, immunologic, and weight-regulating effects of the microbiome likely influence the course and prognosis of this often chronic disease.[5–8] In this article, the authors present the current state of research regarding the interactions between gut microbes and the host organism and initial findings from patients with AN in order to present future directions for AN research and potential treatment options (**Fig. 1**).

MICROBIOME AND BODY WEIGHT REGULATION

It was demonstrated in 2005 that obese patients had a different gut microbiome than normal weight controls.[9] Transplanting stool from obese mice into germ-free (GF) mice that were born and raised in sterile surroundings led to obesity, proving a causal role of gut microbiota in weight regulation.[10] This effect was explained by the ability of certain species of gut microbes in obese individuals to extract more energy from the same amount of food than the gut microbes of lean individuals.[11] Mörkl and colleagues[12] found, for example, that abundance of *Bacteroidetes* species correlated with body mass index in underweight, normal weight, and overweight participants. Three studies so far have shown that *Bacteroidetes* is reduced in underweight patients with AN[6,8,13] and normalized during weight rehabilitation.[8] Further proof for a causal role of the microbiome in body weight regulation comes from Smith and colleagues.[14] They transferred stool from Malawian children with kwashiorkor into GF mice. When fed a Malawian-style diet, the mice developed weight loss and signs of malnutrition, which was not the case in control animals after stool transplantation from nonaffected children. Furthermore, 1 week of treatment with oral antibiotics was able to significantly improve the nutritional status of underweight Malawian children.[15] Compared with stool transfer from waiting-list obese patients, stool transfer from patients who underwent bariatric surgery into GF mice led to a significantly reduced fat mass in mice.[16] As mentioned above and further elaborated later, the microbiome in AN patients also appears to be altered, potentially influencing their metabolization of nutrients and ability to gain weight. Mack and colleagues[8] were able to show significantly differing alterations between restrictive and binge-purging subtypes of AN. Among others factors, this result could be related to the finding that restrictive AN patients need substantially more calories for the same amount of weight gain than their binge-purging AN counterparts.[17]

MICROBIOME AND HORMONAL CHANGES

Microbial changes appear to be associated with hormonal changes in the host; however, this interaction seems to be bidirectional. Although most species of gut microbiota react to host hormones, quite a few can secrete hormonally active substances and influence host hormone secretion.[3] GF mice, for example, showed a 25% higher thyrotropin level[18] and reduced plasma serotonin[19] and catecholamine[20] concentrations relative to those in control mice. Certain gut microbiota produce serotonin,[21] dopamine,[21] and GABA.[20] Estrogen has been shown to decrease bacterial virulence and increase growth rates of certain bacteria in culture[21] and to be correlated with bacterial diversity.[22] Ghrelin, a hormone that increases during fasting, was associated with a higher abundance of *Bacteroides* and *Prevotella* and lower abundances of *Bifidobacterium* and *Lactobacillus* in rats,[23] whereas the satiety hormone leptin showed an inverse association with lower abundance of *Bacteroides* and *Prevotella* and higher abundance of *Bifidobacterium* and *Lactobacillus*. Because AN patients have long-lasting estrogen deficits and amenorrhea, reduced leptin and thyroxin levels, and increased ghrelin levels, a hormonal interaction with the microbiome can be assumed. GF mice were also shown to have increased levels of corticosterone,[24] whereas administration of *Lactobacillus* and *Bifidobacteria* reduced levels of circulating corticoid hormones in rats and humans alike,[25] underlining the role of the gut microbiome in stress regulation. AN patients have repeatedly been found to have increased serum, salivary, and urinary cortisol levels.[26]

MICROBIOME AND GUT PERMEABILITY

Elevated cortisol and stress levels, however, also lead to increased gut permeability.[27] Relatively benign stress, such as speaking publicly, was shown to raise cortisol and intestinal permeability.[28] Potential mechanisms could be the activation of mast cells that carry high-affinity receptors for corticotropin-releasing hormone.[27] In AN, starvation-related stress and increased cortisol could thus lead to enhanced intestinal permeability. In an initial study with AN patients, Mörkl and colleagues[29] did not find any changes in blood zonulin levels, a commonly applied marker for gut permeability.[30,31] Initial animal research results, however, seem to support this hypothesis, as Jesus and colleagues[32] indeed showed a "leaky gut" with an increased colonic permeability, reduced gastric wall thickness, and less tight junction proteins in an AN animal model. This leakiness did not apply to the small intestine, which is in line with research in AN patients that showed a decreased permeability of radioactive-labeled dextran, which is mostly absorbed in the small intestine.[33] Furthermore, there is growing evidence that the gut microbiome also influences gut mucosal barrier function.[34] Colonic permeability in AN could be compromised by certain gut bacteria that preferably digest proteins, including the intestinal mucus, which normally protects the gastric epithelium. Indeed, initial studies in AN showed an increased number of mucin-degrading *Firmicutes* and *Verrucomicrobia*, whereas carbohydrate-degrading taxa and *Bacteroidetes* were less common.[6,8]

MICROBIOME AND INFLAMMATION

Reduced mucin, thinned intestinal walls, and altered tight junctions, all leading to increased intestinal permeability, have been shown to facilitate the translocation of bacterial components, bacterial products, or even complete bacteria across the intestinal wall barrier.[8,32] All three have been shown to trigger immune responses and inflammation,[35-37] potentially via toll-like receptors (TLR-4) triggering proinflammatory cytokine release.[37] AN patients indeed showed increased low-grade inflammation with elevated inflammatory markers, such as tumor necrosis factor-alpha (TNF-α) and interleukin-6 (IL-6) in a recent meta-analysis,[38] in addition to IL-1β from a previous meta-analysis.[39] Animal models of AN confirmed the participation of TLR-4 in releasing mucosal proinflammatory cytokines, and TLR-4 even influenced the animal mortality.[40] Certain *Bifidobacteria*, on the other hand, were able to prevent TLR activation,[41] and *Lactobacilli* were able to reduce TNF-α, IL-6, and IL-8 production.[42] The microbiome thus seems to play an important role in intestinal permeability and inflammation, probably leading to interesting potential treatment options to reduce chronic inflammation in AN.

MICROBIOME AND IMMUNOLOGY

Apart from nonspecific inflammation, bacteria and bacterial subcomponents also induce specific humoral antibodies when traversing the gut barrier. These antibodies can lead to cross-reactivity with body tissue, causing autoimmune diseases that are indeed increased in patients with AN. A large Finnish population cohort study showed elevated odds ratios (ORs) for autoimmune diseases, especially regarding endocrine diseases (OR 2.4) and gastrointestinal diseases (OR 1.8), with Crohn disease being 3.9 times more common in AN patients than in controls.[43] Remarkably, a case study of a Crohn patient who also had AN reported improvement of AN symptoms after receiving anti-TNF-α therapy for Crohn disease. Cross-reactivity of traversing gut bacteria has also led to antibodies against hormones influencing hunger and satiety, such as ghrelin and alpha-melanocyte stimulation hormone (α-MSH).[44] Here, a specific bacterial antigen (ClpB), a part of certain *Enterobacteriaceae*, was actively used to induce antibody formation cross-reactive with α-MSH by injecting it into the animal. The respective *Escherichia coli* species given orally had a similar effect, whereas ClpB-deficient *E coli* did not.[45] Both animal cohorts also showed alterations in food intake and weight regulation, underscoring the functional relevance of these antibodies.[45] A potential mechanism is that cross-reactive antibodies may protect these peptides from degradation in circulation as was shown for ghrelin antibodies.[46] Indeed, in a small group of eating-disordered patients, including patients with AN, increased levels of ClpB were found and were strongly correlated with α-MSH antibodies.[47] Furthermore, eating-disordered patients showed elevated levels of autoantibody to several hunger and satiety-related hormones and α-MSH–reactive antibodies, which in turn correlated with eating-disorder symptom severity.[45] Autoantibodies could thus also be a potential mechanism by which the gut microbiome influences the brain and complex behaviors, such as hunger and satiety, as part of the gut-brain axis.

MICROBIOME AND THE BRAIN (GUT-BRAIN AXIS)

The interactive relationship between the (gut) microbiome and physical development in general and that of the brain specifically becomes apparent in our first moments in life. Whether we were born vaginally or via cesarean section and whether we were breast fed or not determine which different bacteria we come into contact with and have long-lasting influences on our microbiome and our immune system.[48] GF mice with no contact at all with (gut) bacteria showed deviant brain development[49] and altered brain-derived neurotropic factor (BDNF) in the blood and the brain, especially in the hippocampus.[50] BDNF is a neural growth factor responsible for neuron growth, protection, and synapse formation as well as synapse connectivity. Acutely ill AN patients showed reduced serum levels of BDNF, whereas weight recovery seemed to foster normalization.[51] Antibiotics reduced BDNF in the hippocampus of young mice and interestingly also led to increased anxiety levels, demonstrating a direct interaction among the microbiome, brain, and behavior. This interaction becomes even more apparent when considering serotonin metabolism in GF mice, where hippocampal levels of serotonin metabolites 5-hydroxyindoleacetic acid (5-HIAA) and 5-hydroxytryptamine were significantly higher than those seen in normal mice. 5-HIAA was significantly lower in the cerebral spiral fluid of acute AN patients, whereas recovered patients showed higher levels than controls. In addition, peripheral serotonin appeared to be influenced by the gut microbiome via altered number and functioning of enterochromaffin cells in the gut epithelium, leading to stronger peristalsis and thus lower stool transit time; a lack of serotonin-producing microbiota could thus be partially responsible for the often noted obstipation in AN. These nonnegligible amounts of serotonin also enter the bloodstream. Anxiety and depressive symptoms are associated with serotonin metabolism, and both are common comorbidities in AN.[52] The brains of AN patients also showed an extensive loss of gray and white matter volume[53] that was linked to neuropsychological deficits and negative prognosis.[54] The authors' group showed a reduced learning rate for novel objects[55] and reduced cell neogenesis in the brain in an animal model of AN. In a study by Möhle and colleagues[56] in mice, eradication of gut bacteria with antibiotics also led to reduced learning rates and reduced hippocampal cell neogenesis implicating immune processes; supplementation with *Lactobacilli* and *Bifidobacteria* reversed these impairments. Further mechanisms of gut-brain interactions, however, remain to be uncovered.

MICROBIOME IN ANOREXIA NERVOSA

Five cross-sectional studies[13,29,57–59] with 9 to 18 AN patients each and 3 longitudinal studies including 3 to 44 patients[6,8,60] so far have investigated gut microbiome–related changes using stool samples in AN with heterogeneous results.[5,61,62] Kleiman and colleagues[6] and Mörkl and colleagues[29] showed reduced α diversity (a measure of the number of different species in the sample) in acutely ill patients with AN when compared with healthy controls, whereas Mack and colleagues[8] and Borgo and colleagues[58] showed nonsignificant changes in the same direction. Reduced α diversity is observed in obese patients and patients with inflammatory bowel disease and associated with increased gut permeability and inflammation levels.[63] Mack and colleagues[8] showed a significant increase in α diversity following weight rehabilitation, and Kleiman and colleagues reported a similar trend. Interestingly, in Kleiman and colleagues' sample, diversity was correlated with depression scores and eating disorder symptoms. β-Diversity (a measure of the microbiome similarity between different individuals) was found to be higher in Mack and colleagues' and Kleiman and colleagues' samples, evidencing more heterogeneity in AN patients. Although β-diversity also decreased during weight gain, AN patients' microbiome still differed significantly from that of healthy controls, more closely resembling their own microbiome during acute starvation. This result hints at enduring changes in the microbiome of AN patients even after short-term weight recovery. Regarding specific species abundances, *Firmicutes* were increased and *Bacteroidetes* were reduced in the sample of Mack and colleagues, and a similar trend was found in Kleiman and colleagues' sample. A reduced number of *Roseburia* species were found in 2 study samples,[8,58] and increased numbers of the methane-producing archaeon *Methanobrevibacter smithii* were found in 3 samples.[8,57,58] The latter was found to inversely correlate with body mass index[57] and could represent an adaptive mechanism to increase energy exploitation.[8] The relative increase in *Firmicutes* could potentially further raise gut permeability, because it degrades mostly proteins, including gut mucin. Reduced *Roseburia*, on the other hand, feeds on carbohydrates and normally produces butyrate. Butyrate has previously been shown to reduce intestinal permeability[64] and inflammation[65]; its absence would thus further promote these phenomena. Furthermore, Mack and colleagues[8] and Morita and colleagues[59] showed increased levels of branched-chain fatty acids, fermentation products of protein degradation that have been shown to further support peptide YY production, a gastric peptide that negatively affects appetite and increases depressiveness.[66]

DISCUSSION
The Importance of Microbiome Research in Anorexia Nervosa

The human microbiome is rapidly becoming an important research topic in somatic and psychiatric diseases.[4,5,35,63] In AN, the influence of the gut microbiome on food utilization, hunger and satiety, gastrointestinal dysfunction, neurocognitive function, mood, anxiety, and other outcomes needs further intensive research. Underlying pathophysiologic mechanisms, including gut permeability, inflammation, autoantibodies, hormonal interactions, and the gut-brain axis, need to be studied in depth. Longitudinal observation studies regarding microbiome diversity and taxa abundance need to map starvation-induced changes and potential rehabilitation or persisting deviations in AN patients. Also, current refeeding regimens for AN patients should be questioned, if the regimen does not take potential interactions with the gut microbiome into account. AN patients often eat vegetarian or vegan diets low in fat and carbohydrates and high in protein and fiber before therapy. Upon refeeding, this pattern changes dramatically, because hospital food is mostly high in calories and rich in carbohydrates and fat. In addition, patients requiring oral supplements or nasogastric feeding mostly receive products based on cow's milk. Animal-based foods have been shown to rapidly change the abundance of particular microbial species when previously maintained on a vegetarian diet[67] and might increase certain inflammation-inducing bacteria.[5] Further preclinical and clinical research on the effect of refeeding on the gut microbiome is needed to evaluate and improve current methods of refeeding in AN. Intervention trials using psychobiotics ("live bacteria, which when applied in adequate amounts, confer mental health benefits"[35]), prebiotics (dietary fibers furthering the growth of these positive bacteria), nutritional supplements, and nutritional interventions (eg, vegan/vegetarian/nonvegetarian food) need to be conducted. Preclinical research shows promising health benefits,[34] for example, regarding mood and cognitive functioning in healthy adults,[68,69] and initial positive results also for mental disorders.[70] Pirbaglou and colleagues[71] recently published a systematic review of 10 randomized controlled trials regarding the use of psychobiotics against anxiety and depression in patients. The investigators summarized the preliminary evidence they found in the detection of psychological benefits from psychobiotics while suggesting methodological limitations regarding the heterogeneous use of different bacterial strains. However, so far, no intervention study regarding AN has been published.

MICROBIOME IN ANOREXIA NERVOSA THERAPY

Microbiome-directed interventions could thus become an important addition to the current treatment of AN patients. There are several different mechanisms by which these interventions could be administered, as follows:

- Nutritional supply itself
- Nutritional supplements
- Probiotics (live bacteria)
- Prebiotics (fibers favoring growth of certain bacteria)
- Drugs influencing the microbiome[72]

Therapeutic goals could be identified at different levels of the microbiome-host interaction in AN patients:

- Induction of increased energy retrieval from the same amount of food to increase weight gain while not increasing food volume

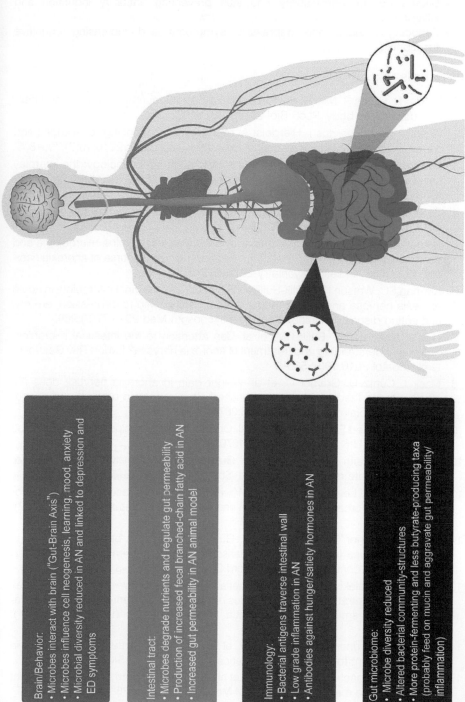

Brain/Behavior:
• Microbes interact with brain ("Gut-Brain Axis")
• Microbes influence cell neogenesis, learning, mood, anxiety
• Microbial diversity reduced in AN and linked to depression and ED symptoms

Intestinal tract:
• Microbes degrade nutrients and regulate gut permeability
• Production of increased fecal branched-chain fatty acid in AN
• Increased gut permeability in AN animal model

Immunology:
• Bacterial antigens traverse intestinal wall
• Low grade inflammation in AN
• Antibodies against hunger/satiety hormones in AN

Gut microbiome:
• Microbe diversity reduced
• Altered bacterial community-structures
• More protein-fermenting and less butyrate-producing taxa (probably feed on mucin and aggravate gut permeability/inflammation)

Fig. 1. Gut microbiome interactions in patients with AN.

- Decreasing gut permeability and thus preventing antibody induction and inflammation
- Reducing anxious and depressive symptoms and increasing cognitive functioning

REFERENCES

1. Sender R, Fuchs S, Milo R. Revised estimates for the number of human and bacteria cells in the body. PLoS Biol 2016;14(8):e1002533.
2. Clavel T, Lagkouvardos I, Hiergeist A. Microbiome sequencing: challenges and opportunities for molecular medicine. Expert Rev Mol Diagn 2016;16(7):795–805.
3. Neuman H, Debelius JW, Knight R, et al. Microbial endocrinology: the interplay between the microbiota and the endocrine system. FEMS Microbiol Rev 2015; 39(4):509–21.
4. Cryan JF, Dinan TG. Mind-altering microorganisms: the impact of the gut microbiota on brain and behaviour. Nat Rev Neurosci 2012;13(10):701–12.
5. Herpertz-Dahlmann B, Seitz J, Baines J. Food matters: how the microbiome and gut–brain interaction might impact the development and course of anorexia nervosa. Eur Child Adolesc Psychiatry 2017;26(9):1031–41.
6. Kleiman SC, Watson HJ, Bulik-Sullivan EC, et al. The intestinal microbiota in acute anorexia nervosa and during renourishment: relationship to depression, anxiety, and eating disorder psychopathology. Psychosom Med 2015;77(9):969.
7. Carr J, Kleiman SC, Bulik CM, et al. Can attention to the intestinal microbiota improve understanding and treatment of anorexia nervosa? Expert Rev Gastroenterol Hepatol 2016;10(5):565–9.
8. Mack I, Cuntz U, Grämer C, et al. Weight gain in anorexia nervosa does not ameliorate the faecal microbiota, branched chain fatty acid profiles, and gastrointestinal complaints. Sci Rep 2016;6:26752.
9. Ley RE, Bäckhed F, Turnbaugh P, et al. Obesity alters gut microbial ecology. Proc Natl Acad Sci U S A 2005;102(31):11070–5.
10. Ridaura VK, Faith JJ, Rey FE, et al. Gut microbiota from twins discordant for obesity modulate metabolism in mice. Science 2013;341(6150):1241214.
11. Turnbaugh PJ, Ley RE, Mahowald MA, et al. An obesity-associated gut microbiome with increased capacity for energy harvest. Nature 2006;444(7122): 1027–31.
12. Mörkl S, Lackner S, Müller W, et al. Gut microbiota and body composition in anorexia nervosa inpatients in comparison to athletes, overweight, obese, and normal weight controls. Int J Eat Disord 2017;50(12):1421–31.
13. Million M, Angelakis E, Maraninchi M, et al. Correlation between body mass index and gut concentrations of Lactobacillus reuteri, Bifidobacterium animalis, Methanobrevibacter smithii and Escherichia coli. Int J Obes (Lond) 2013;37(11): 1460–6.
14. Smith MI, Yatsunenko T, Manary MJ, et al. Gut microbiomes of Malawian twin pairs discordant for kwashiorkor. Science 2013;339(6119):548–54.
15. Trehan I, Goldbach HS, LaGrone LN, et al. Antibiotics as part of the management of severe acute malnutrition. N Engl J Med 2013;368(5):425–35.
16. Tremaroli V, Karlsson F, Werling M, et al. Roux-en-Y gastric bypass and vertical banded gastroplasty induce long-term changes on the human gut microbiome contributing to fat mass regulation. Cell Metab 2015;22(2):228–38.

17. Marzola E, Nasser JA, Hashim SA, et al. Nutritional rehabilitation in anorexia nervosa: review of the literature and implications for treatment. BMC Psychiatry 2013; 13:290.

18. Wostmann B. Morphology and physiology, endocrinology and biochemistry. In: Wostmann BS, editor. Germfree and gnotobiotic animal models. Boca Raton (FL): CRC Press; 1996. p. 43–71.

19. Wikoff WR, Anfora AT, Liu J, et al. Metabolomics analysis reveals large effects of gut microflora on mammalian blood metabolites. Proc Natl Acad Sci U S A 2009; 106(10):3698–703.

20. Asano Y, Hiramoto T, Nishino R, et al. Critical role of gut microbiota in the production of biologically active, free catecholamines in the gut lumen of mice. Am J Physiol Gastrointest Liver Physiol 2012;303(11):G1288–95.

21. Roshchina V. Evolutionary considerations of neurotransmitters in microbial, plant, and animal cells. In: Lyte M, Fitzgerald P, editors. Microbial endocrinology: interkingdom signaling in infectious disease and health. New York: Springer; 2010. p. 17–52.

22. Flores R, Shi J, Fuhrman B, et al. Fecal microbial determinants of fecal and systemic estrogens and estrogen metabolites: a cross-sectional study. J Transl Med 2012;10:253.

23. Queipo-Ortuño MI, Seoane LM, Murri M, et al. Gut microbiota composition in male rat models under different nutritional status and physical activity and its association with serum leptin and ghrelin levels. PLoS One 2013;8(5):e65465.

24. Grenham S, Clarke G, Cryan JF, et al. Brain-gut-microbe communication in health and disease. Front Physiol 2011;2:94.

25. Messaoudi M, Lalonde R, Violle N, et al. Assessment of psychotropic-like properties of a probiotic formulation (Lactobacillus helveticus R0052 and Bifidobacterium longum R0175) in rats and human subjects. Br J Nutr 2011;105(5):755–64.

26. Schorr M, Miller KK. The endocrine manifestations of anorexia nervosa: mechanisms and management. Nat Rev Endocrinol 2017;13(3):174–86.

27. Petra AI, Panagiotidou S, Stewart JM, et al. Spectrum of mast cell activation disorders. Expert Rev Clin Immunol 2014;10(6):729–39.

28. Vanuytsel T, van Wanrooy S, Vanheel H, et al. Psychological stress and corticotropin-releasing hormone increase intestinal permeability in humans by a mast cell-dependent mechanism. Gut 2014;63(8):1293–9.

29. Mörkl S, Lackner S, Meinitzer A, et al. Pilot study: gut microbiome and intestinal barrier in anorexia nervosa. Fortschr Neurol Psychiatr 2018. https://doi.org/10. 1055/s-0043-123826 [in German].

30. Fasano A, Not T, Wang W, et al. Zonulin, a newly discovered modulator of intestinal permeability, and its expression in coeliac disease. Lancet Lond Engl 2000; 355(9214):1518–9.

31. Sturgeon C, Fasano A. Zonulin, a regulator of epithelial and endothelial barrier functions, and its involvement in chronic inflammatory diseases. Tissue Barriers 2016;4(4):e1251384.

32. Jesus P, Ouelaa W, Francois M, et al. Alteration of intestinal barrier function during activity-based anorexia in mice. Clin Nutr 2014;33(6):1046–53.

33. Monteleone P, Carratù R, Cartenì M, et al. Intestinal permeability is decreased in anorexia nervosa. Mol Psychiatry 2004;9(1):76–80.

34. Kelly JR, Kennedy PJ, Cryan JF, et al. Breaking down the barriers: the gut microbiome, intestinal permeability and stress-related psychiatric disorders. Front Cell Neurosci 2015;9:392.

35. Dinan TG, Stanton C, Cryan JF. Psychobiotics: a novel class of psychotropic. Biol Psychiatry 2013;74(10):720–6.
36. Kelly JR, Minuto C, Cryan JF, et al. Cross talk: the microbiota and neurodevelopmental disorders. Front Neurosci 2017;11:490.
37. Bambury A, Sandhu K, Cryan JF, et al. Finding the needle in the haystack: systematic identification of psychobiotics. Br J Pharmacol 2017. https://doi.org/10.1111/bph.14127.
38. Dalton B, Bartholdy S, Robinson L, et al. A meta-analysis of cytokine concentrations in eating disorders. J Psychiatr Res 2018;103:252–64.
39. Solmi M, Veronese N, Favaro A, et al. Inflammatory cytokines and anorexia nervosa: a meta-analysis of cross-sectional and longitudinal studies. Psychoneuroendocrinology 2015;51:237–52.
40. Belmonte L, Achamrah N, Nobis S, et al. A role for intestinal TLR4-driven inflammatory response during activity-based anorexia. Sci Rep 2016;6:35813.
41. Zhou W, Lv H, Li MX, et al. Protective effects of bifidobacteria on intestines in newborn rats with necrotizing enterocolitis and its regulation on TLR2 and TLR4. Genet Mol Res 2015;14(3):11505–14.
42. Dai C, Zheng C-Q, Meng F-J, et al. VSL#3 probiotics exerts the anti-inflammatory activity via PI3k/Akt and NF-κB pathway in rat model of DSS-induced colitis. Mol Cell Biochem 2013;374(1–2):1–11.
43. Raevuori A, Haukka J, Vaarala O, et al. The increased risk for autoimmune diseases in patients with eating disorders. PLoS One 2014;9(8):e104845.
44. Fetissov SO. Role of the gut microbiota in host appetite control: bacterial growth to animal feeding behaviour. Nat Rev Endocrinol 2017;13(1):11.
45. Tennoune N, Chan P, Breton J, et al. Bacterial ClpB heat-shock protein, an antigen-mimetic of the anorexigenic peptide alpha-MSH, at the origin of eating disorders. Transl Psychiatry 2014;4:e458.
46. François M, Barde S, Legrand R, et al. High-fat diet increases ghrelin-expressing cells in stomach, contributing to obesity. Nutrition 2016;32(6):709–15.
47. Breton J, Legrand R, Akkermann K, et al. Elevated plasma concentrations of bacterial ClpB protein in patients with eating disorders. Int J Eat Disord 2016;49(8):805–8.
48. Santoro A, Ostan R, Candela M, et al. Gut microbiota changes in the extreme decades of human life: a focus on centenarians. Cell Mol Life Sci 2018;75(1):129–48.
49. Luczynski P, McVey Neufeld K-A, Oriach CS, et al. Growing up in a bubble: using germ-free animals to assess the influence of the gut microbiota on brain and behavior. Int J Neuropsychopharmacol 2016;19(8). https://doi.org/10.1007/s00018-017-2674-y.
50. Sherwin E, Rea K, Dinan TG, et al. A gut (microbiome) feeling about the brain. Curr Opin Gastroenterol 2016;32(2):96–102.
51. Zwipp J, Hass J, Schober I, et al. Serum brain-derived neurotrophic factor and cognitive functioning in underweight, weight-recovered and partially weight-recovered females with anorexia nervosa. Prog Neuropsychopharmacol Biol Psychiatry 2014;54:163–9.
52. Herpertz-Dahlmann B. Adolescent eating disorders: update on definitions, symptomatology, epidemiology, and comorbidity. Child Adolesc Psychiatr Clin N Am 2015;24(1):177–96.
53. Seitz J, Herpertz-Dahlmann B, Konrad K. Brain morphological changes in adolescent and adult patients with anorexia nervosa. J Neural Transm 2016;123(8):949–59.

54. Seitz J, Walter M, Mainz V, et al. Brain volume reduction predicts weight develop-
    ment in adolescent patients with anorexia nervosa. J Psychiatr Res 2015;68:228–37.
55. Paulukat L, Frintrop L, Liesbrock J, et al. Memory impairment is associated with
    the loss of regular oestrous cycle and plasma oestradiol levels in an activity-
    based anorexia animal model. World J Biol Psychiatry 2016;17(4):274–84.
56. Möhle L, Mattei D, Heimesaat MM, et al. Ly6Chi monocytes provide a link be-
    tween antibiotic-induced changes in gut microbiota and adult hippocampal neu-
    rogenesis. Cell Rep 2016;15(9):1945–56.
57. Armougom F, Henry M, Vialettes B, et al. Monitoring bacterial community of hu-
    man gut microbiota reveals an increase in Lactobacillus in obese patients and
    Methanogens in anorexic patients. PLoS One 2009;4(9):e7125.
58. Borgo F, Riva A, Benetti A, et al. Microbiota in anorexia nervosa: the triangle be-
    tween bacterial species, metabolites and psychological tests. PLoS One 2017;
    12(6):e0179739.
59. Morita C, Tsuji H, Hata T, et al. Gut dysbiosis in patients with anorexia nervosa.
    PLoS One 2015;10(12):e0145274.
60. Kleiman SC, Glenny EM, Bulik-Sullivan EC, et al. Daily changes in composition
    and diversity of the intestinal microbiota in patients with anorexia nervosa: a se-
    ries of three cases. Eur Eat Disord Rev 2017;25(5):423–7.
61. Mack I, Penders J, Cook J, et al. Is the impact of starvation on the gut microbiota
    specific or unspecific to anorexia nervosa? A narrative review based on a system-
    atic literature search. Curr Neuropharmacol 2018;16(8):1131–49.
62. Seitz J, Baines J, Herpertz-Dahlmann B. Microbiome and inflammation in eating
    disorders. In: Hebebrand J, Herpertz-Dahlmann B, editors. Eating disorders and
    obesity in childhood and adolescence. Philadelphia: Elsevier; in press.
63. Kostic AD, Xavier RJ, Gevers D. The microbiome in inflammatory bowel disease:
    current status and the future ahead. Gastroenterology 2014;146(6):1489–99.
64. Geirnaert A, Calatayud M, Grootaert C, et al. Butyrate-producing bacteria supple-
    mented in vitro to Crohn's disease patient microbiota increased butyrate produc-
    tion and enhanced intestinal epithelial barrier integrity. Sci Rep 2017;7(1):11450.
65. Vieira AT, Fukumori C, Ferreira CM. New insights into therapeutic strategies for
    gut microbiota modulation in inflammatory diseases. Clin Transl Immunology
    2016;5(6):e87.
66. Holzer P, Farzi A. Neuropeptides and the microbiota-gut-brain axis. Adv Exp Med
    Biol 2014;817:195–219.
67. David LA, Maurice CF, Carmody RN, et al. Diet rapidly and reproducibly alters the
    human gut microbiome. Nature 2014;505(7484):559–63.
68. Bagga D, Reichert JL, Koschutnig K, et al. Probiotics drive gut microbiome trig-
    gering emotional brain signatures. Gut Microbes 2018;9(6):486–96.
69. Bagga D, Aigner CS, Reichert JL, et al. Influence of 4-week multi-strain probiotic
    administration on resting-state functional connectivity in healthy volunteers. Eur J
    Nutr 2018. [Epub ahead of print].
70. Kelly JR, Allen AP, Temko A, et al. Lost in translation? The potential psychobiotic
    Lactobacillus rhamnosus (JB-1) fails to modulate stress or cognitive performance
    in healthy male subjects. Brain Behav Immun 2017;61:50–9.
71. Pirbaglou M, Katz J, de Souza RJ, et al. Probiotic supplementation can positively
    affect anxiety and depressive symptoms: a systematic review of randomized
    controlled trials. Nutr Res 2016;36(9):889–98.
72. Maier L, Pruteanu M, Kuhn M, et al. Extensive impact of non-antibiotic drugs on
    human gut bacteria. Nature 2018;555(7698):623.

Personality Variables and Eating Pathology

Allison F. Wagner, MA*, Kelly M. Vitousek, PhD

KEYWORDS

- Eating disorders • Anorexia nervosa • Bulimia nervosa • Personality • Perfectionism
- Impulsivity

KEY POINTS

- Specific features of the eating disorders must be considered when interpreting personality data, including starvation effects, frequent crossover between diagnostic categories, the low stability of personality pathology in young and acutely ill patients, and the Persistence of residual symptoms as well as scarring effects in recovered samples.
- The temperamental dimensions of Harm Avoidance and Neuroticism represent broad vulnerability factors for many psychiatric disorders; scores are elevated across eating disorder diagnoses and tend to reduce but not normalize with recovery. High levels of Novelty Seeking are associated with binge-eating and purging; low Novelty Seeking and elevated Persistence characterize patients with restricting anorexia nervosa.
- Exceptionally high scores on indices of both negative and positive perfectionism are characteristic of eating disorders and may be related to distinctive beliefs about the value of symptoms.
- Negative urgency is a strong predictor of bulimic behaviors; however, episodes do not reflect a pervasive pattern of impulsivity in all patients who binge eat.
- Empirically derived personality prototypes may predict risk factors, comorbidity, and outcome better than specific eating disorder diagnoses.

The psychological features of eating disorders (EDs) are linked in multiple and reciprocal ways to most of the topic areas summarized in this issue. Genetic risk is encoded, in part, through temperamental traits that increase the likelihood of developing anorexia nervosa (AN) or bulimia nervosa (BN) (see Cynthia M. Bulik and colleagues' article, "Genetics of Eating Disorders: What the Clinician Needs to Know," in this issue), especially within a sociocultural context that promotes control over eating and weight (see Siân A. McLean and Susan J. Paxton's article, "Body Image

Disclosure Statement: The authors have no potential conflicts of interest or financial disclosures.
Department of Psychology, University of Hawai'i at Mānoa, 2530 Dole Street, Sakamaki C400, Honolulu, HI 96826, USA
* Corresponding author.
E-mail address: afwagner@hawaii.edu

Psychiatr Clin N Am 42 (2019) 105–119
https://doi.org/10.1016/j.psc.2018.10.012
0193-953X/19/© 2018 Elsevier Inc. All rights reserved.

in the Context of Eating Disorders,"; and Ruth Striegel Weissman's article, "The Role of Sociocultural Factors in the Etiology of Eating Disorders," in this issue). Diagnostic criteria specify characteristic attitudes about the body and the self, as well as characteristic eating and weight control behaviors (see B. Timothy Walsh's article, "Diagnostic Categories for Eating Disorders: Current Status and What Lies Ahead," in this issue). The high rate and pattern of comorbidity mirror trait profiles in ED subgroups; in fact, some findings suggest that subtyping on the basis of personality features may be more useful than conferring specific ED diagnoses according to current symptom picture. The methods of cognitive neuroscience are yielding new information and different perspectives on key personality variables such as impulsivity and perseverance (see Joanna E. Steinglass and colleagues' article, "Cognitive Neuroscience of Eating Disorders," in this issue). Biological aspects of EDs are so intertwined with psychological elements that both are distorted when considered in isolation from one another (see Joanna E. Steinglass and colleagues' article, "Cognitive Neuroscience of Eating Disorders,"; and Jochen Seitz and colleagues' article, "The Microbiome and Eating Disorders," in this issue).

The close relationship between biological and psychological aspects makes it challenging to identify the boundaries of a pure review of temperamental variables in EDs. This summary focuses principally on personality variables assessed through self-report and structured interviews, with abbreviated discussions of other topic areas and measurement techniques. It should be remembered throughout, however, that consideration of psychological elements cannot be detached from the context provided by the accompanying reviews.

PERSONALITY TRAITS AND DISORDERS
Prominence in Clinical Descriptions and Causal Models

Personality variables have been invoked to account for AN throughout its recorded history, with striking consistency across observers and over time. In the middle of the past century, for example, the typical anorexic patient was described as rigid, driven, hyperconscientious, insecure, sensitive, and introverted—a "rank perfectionist ... (who lacks) the warmth and spontaneity that are consistent with her years."[1(p109)] Diverse theoretical models, from the psychodynamic to the cognitive-behavioral, implicate this cluster of traits in the development and maintenance of the disorder, as well as its resistance to treatment.

After BN was recognized in the late 1970s, temperamental factors also figured prominently in efforts to explain symptom divergence. Observers hypothesized that individuals who shared numerous risk factors and eating/weight concerns might be shaped in different behavioral directions partly through the influence of other premorbid personality traits. It was conjectured that those with higher levels of impulsivity and affective instability would find it more difficult to sustain dietary restraint than individuals with a stronger loading of compulsive traits and would be both more susceptible to and in need of the emotion-regulating effects of binge-purge episodes.

The assumption that specific personality variables had pathoplastic effects on symptom expression in these related but discriminable disorders[2] provided much of the impetus for research in this area. Nonetheless, early investigators were already struck by the heterogeneity they observed within as well as between diagnostic categories,[3,4] cautioning that an exclusive focus on the bulimic-restricting dimension oversimplified the complex clinical picture presented by both disorders and belied the substantial overlap and frequent crossover between them.[5] Successive reviews have affirmed similar conclusions for the past 25 years.[6–12] Using larger samples, better measures, and more rigorous designs, data from hundreds of studies have refined initial impressions of personality variables in AN, BN, and binge-eating disorder (BED), while continuing to highlight the same clusters of traits as probable contributors to the onset, maintenance, and form of EDs.

Assessment Challenges in Eating Disorder Populations

Methodological and interpretive problems abound across all efforts to elucidate relationships between personality and psychopathology, which can interact in a variety of ways.[9,12] Prospective designs are needed to establish the temporal precedence of traits as putative risk factors; however, such endeavors can yield scanty returns at extraordinary expense, particularly for low base-rate disorders. In most of the small set of longitudinal studies in the ED field, too few full-syndrome cases have emerged to permit the identification of predisposing traits for AN or BN, although some psychological variables have been linked to subthreshold symptoms.

The bulk of the available evidence has been assembled through cross-sectional designs that share significant, and in some instances irremediable, limitations.[5,9,13,14] The most obvious is that assessors must infer dimensions of a patient's "usual self" from data gathered when he or she is acutely symptomatic, although "this is perhaps the worst time to do so."[2(p103)] When individuals who are cycling unhappily between dieting, binge eating, and purging characterize themselves as "impulsive," "dysregulated," or "ineffective," it is impossible to determine whether they are describing stable predilections that preceded and perhaps prompted their ED symptoms or are reporting their views of themselves in the throes of BN. Other problems include: the low stability of personality pathology over time, particularly in adolescents; inflated estimates of disturbance based on self-report versus clinician-rated scales; sampling biases when cases are drawn from intensive treatment settings rather than the full range of affected individuals; and the omission of appropriate comparison groups, such as psychiatric and/or dieting controls. In addition, efforts to consolidate the accumulating data are hampered by construct overlap across different inventories of temperamental traits and personality characteristics.[15] Multiple terms have been created to label highly similar or closely related variables such as Novelty Seeking, sensation seeking, and impulsivity, which are sometimes construed as fundamental elements of temperament and sometimes as partly state-dependent phenomena influenced by learning history and current context.

Specific features of EDs compound the challenge of personality assessment in the general case.[5,8,16] The behavior of normal humans and animals is profoundly and predictably altered by food deprivation,[17,18] making it difficult to disentangle the state effects of starvation and chaotic eating from traits that may induce individuals to restrict. The consistency of these changes across species, individuals, and conditions suggests that most represent adaptive responses to the stress of starvation, selected because they reduce energy expenditure and/or focus the organism's attention on securing food. Accounts of human starvation repeatedly allude to the sense that its victims undergo a startling change in "personality," becoming depressed, irritable, perseverative, self-centered, socially withdrawn, and sexually indifferent.[17]

The collection of data from remitted patients with ED can be used both to document and mitigate these confounding effects. Personality pathology is generally attenuated in recovered samples compared with patients with active EDs, whereas some disturbances persist relative to healthy controls. Although these profiles almost certainly approximate stable functioning better than data obtained from individuals who are starving or eating erratically, the assumption that post-treatment assessment recaptures premorbid status is unjustified. Personality patterns measured after remission are likely to represent an unknown blend of enduring traits, residual ED symptoms, "scars" of previous illness, and treatment effects. Moreover, fully recovered samples cannot be considered a representative subset of the patient population as a whole, especially in the case of severe, refractory disorders such as AN.

Another set of challenges relate to the classification of ED subtypes. Some of these problems are technical, such as discrepancies in the way groups have been formed and reported as diagnostic criteria evolve and/or at investigators' discretion. Data from AN patients who fit the restricting (ANR) and binge-purge (ANBP) subtypes are sometimes analyzed separately and sometimes combined; subthreshold cases with other specified feeding or eating disorders (OSFED) (formerly ED not otherwise specified [EDNOS]) may be examined as a group, allocated to the best-matching full-syndrome category, or excluded.

Other problems are linked to more fundamental conceptual and classification issues that carry important, and bidirectional, implications for personality research. As noted earlier, it has been evident for decades that ED diagnostic subgroups are indistinct, heterogeneous, and unstable. Individuals assigned to different categories on the basis of weight status and the presence/absence of binge eating and purging behaviors share not only central elements of ED psychopathology but several common personality features. At the same time, markedly different personality profiles can be discerned within each diagnostic group, in some cases matching the prototypic features hypothesized to shape symptom expression for that category and in others suggesting a different ED subtype; for example, impulsivity and emotional dysregulation are prominent in a subset of patients with AN, whereas obsessionality and constraint characterize some of those with BN. In addition, crossover between ED categories is substantial, with estimates ranging from 38% to 64% for movement from ANR to ANB and from 7% to 54% for transition from AN to BN; shifts toward restriction and subnormal weight occur more rarely.[19–21] The fact that a single patient may be diagnosed in turn with ANR, ANBP, and BN over the course of a continuous ED violates the principles of psychiatric classification and argues for more inclusive, transdiagnostic models of ED psychopathology.[22] It also poses significant problems for personality research. For example, when data from individuals with AN who are passing through a transient phase of restriction before binge eating develops are combined with data from those with stable ANR, any associations that may exist between personality traits and diagnostic subtype are inevitably weakened.[5]

Dimensions of Temperament

Broadband or multiscale measures of personality are designed to assess basic elements of temperament that are biologically based, moderately heritable, apparent early in life, and fairly stable across contexts.[23] Much of the recent ED research has derived from Cloninger's[24] psychobiological model, which was revised to include four dimensions of temperament (Harm Avoidance, Novelty Seeking, Persistence, and Reward Dependence) as well as 3 "character" dimensions posited to develop through experience and to interact with temperament to influence the emergence of psychopathology. Inventories based on Digman's[25] five-factor model, measuring Neuroticism, Extraversion, Openness, Agreeableness, and Conscientiousness, have also been used extensively.

Descriptive and meta-analytic reviews indicate that all ED subgroups score high on Harm Avoidance compared with healthy controls, indicating propensities for excessive worry, fear of uncertainty, and behavioral inhibition to avoid the possibility of punishment.[6–9,26] This pattern corresponds with high Neuroticism and low Extraversion scores on five-factor inventories[8] and is consonant with retrospective reports describing anorexic and bulimic individuals as anxious and obsessive-compulsive in childhood.[27–29] Elevated scores tend to abate but not normalize after ED symptoms resolve.[6,30,31] Harm Avoidance and Neuroticism are considered broad vulnerability factors for most psychiatric disorders, so that the prominence of these features in patients with ED cannot be construed as a hallmark for eating and weight pathology. In fact, a meta-analytic review found that individuals with AN, BN, and alcohol use disorders had significantly lower elevations on Harm Avoidance than all other psychiatric comparison groups with the exception of bipolar disorder.[26]

If Harm Avoidance and Neuroticism are common to varied forms of psychopathology, several dimensions of temperament differentiate diagnostic categories within the EDs. Binge eating subgroups, particularly BN, show high levels of Novelty Seeking compared with healthy controls, suggesting a propensity for impulsive decision-making and behavioral activation in response to new stimuli and potential reward; in contrast, individuals with AN obtain lower than average scores on this index. Data from other psychiatric groups indicate that Novelty Seeking is also elevated in patients with substance use disorders, bipolar disorder, and cluster B personality disorders. Patients with AN are characterized by higher levels of Persistence than normal controls, indicating a tendency toward sustained, diligent effort despite frustration or intermittent reward. Other ED groups also score relatively high on this factor, although Persistence is significantly more elevated in restricting AN samples than groups with BN, BED, or OSFED (formerly EDNOS).

Other dimensions of temperament have shown minimal and/or inconsistent associations with ED pathology. Although some models hypothesize a linkage between Reward Dependence and AN,[32] no differences have been demonstrated between AN samples and other ED subgroups or healthy controls on this index of sensitivity to social approval.[6–8,30] Lower scores on the character dimension of Self-Directedness are associated with binge eating and purging behaviors[7,8] and predict diagnostic crossover[21] and poorer long-term outcome in BN samples.[33]

Personality Disorders

The voluminous literature on personality disorders and EDs has been analyzed in numerous reviews[5,7,8,10,16,34,35] and will not be discussed in detail. Rates of comorbidity are typically high but dramatically variable, ranging from 27% to 93% for the presence of any personality disorder in mixed ED samples and from 2% to 47% when specific personality disorder diagnoses are reported for specific EDs. These marked discrepancies stem from the well-known problems posed by categorical versus dimensional assessment, including inconsistent diagnostic procedures and criteria and the instability of personality disorder diagnoses, especially in younger and/or acutely distressed groups. Although the construct of personality disorders depends on the judgment that patterns are characteristic of long-term functioning, more than half of patients with ED who are assigned a personality disorder diagnosis at intake no longer meet criteria when reassessed.

In spite of these limitations, a few relatively consistent conclusions have emerged. Cluster C diagnoses (avoidant, dependent, obsessive compulsive) are frequent in both AN and BN subtypes, reflecting the shared tendencies toward Neuroticism and Harm Avoidance seen on measures of temperament. Consonant with the differential pattern of scores on Persistence and Novelty Seeking, approximately twice as many patients AN as patients with BN are diagnosed with Obsessive Compulsive Personality Disorder (OCPD), whereas the cluster B diagnosis of Borderline Personality Disorder (BPD) is assigned to a somewhat greater proportion of binge-eating subgroups. BPD features more often attenuate below threshold levels as ED symptoms remit, whereas OCPD patterns tend to persist, suggesting that impulsivity and affective instability are especially state-dependent.

MULTIDIMENSIONAL CHARACTERISTICS AND THEIR INTERACTIONS

Across clinical descriptions, theoretical models, and research on personality disorders and dimensions, several themes recur as particularly relevant to understanding EDs. Two that have been investigated intensively are reviewed in more detail below. Perfectionism seems to be a risk factor for developing any ED and may play an important role in maintaining symptoms across ED subtypes, while impulsivity contributes to the form of symptom expression. Both are complex constructs that represent a blend of basic temperamental traits with attitudes, expectancies, values, and habitual behaviors shaped in part by learning history.

Perfectionism

Sketches of the prototypic AN personality have featured perfectionism since the syndrome was first described; more recently, it has been conceptualized as a key maintaining and perhaps initiating mechanism for BN as well.[22,36] It makes intuitive sense that disorders defined by desperate efforts to exert control over eating and weight might be associated with a general disposition to set unrealistic standards and persist in the struggle to achieve them despite escalating costs and frequent failures. Investigators have found it exceptionally difficult, however, to reach consensus on how the complex and context-dependent construct of perfectionism should be operationalized.[37–40] The database on perfectionism and EDs is complicated by the use of alternative models and measures; nonetheless, the unusual pattern of results obtained for this patient population helps to clarify both the nature of perfectionism and the distinctive psychopathology of EDs.

Perfectionism carries simultaneously positive and negative connotations for laypeople and clinicians alike, subsuming elements of both an admirable pursuit of excellence and potentially crippling fears of falling short.[41] Although some measures are unidimensional, such as the widely used Perfectionism subscale of the Eating Disorders Inventory,[42] most were constructed to assess multiple facets and presumed correlates of perfectionism, including high personal standards, concern over mistakes, doubts about actions, perceived pressures for performance, expectations and experiences of criticism, and orderliness or organization.[43,44] Not all of these conceptually linked variables are empirically related, but two constructs repeatedly emerge. One is broadly interpreted as "adaptive," "positive," or "healthy" perfectionism, representing high standard-setting and striving for achievement, while the other is deemed "maladaptive," "negative," "neurotic," or "clinical" perfectionism, including evaluative concerns, self-criticism for error, and perceived pressure from others.[37,39,45] Initial findings in normal samples and most psychiatric groups suggested that only the maladaptive constituents predicted variables such as Neuroticism, depression, low self-esteem, and burnout, whereas high standard-setting is associated with Conscientiousness on five-factor inventories and has few negative correlates. Debate continues about whether achievement striving should be considered a variant of perfectionism at all, with some experts reserving the term for a compulsive pursuit of excessively stringent standards that is motivated by evaluative concerns. More recent evidence, however, indicates that even the ostensibly adaptive aspects of perfectionism are correlated with higher levels of depression[46] and increased suicidal ideation[47]; as noted later, they are also implicated in the psychopathology of EDs.

No matter how the construct is operationalized, individuals with AN and BN obtain high and generally comparable scores on perfectionism measures, typically exceeding both normal and psychiatric comparison groups; less consistent findings are reported for BED.[7,8,37,48] Reviews highlight several lines of evidence suggesting that perfectionism represents a stable trait in this population rather than a consequence of illness: family and twin studies indicate that perfectionism is partly heritable in ED samples; retrospective reports describe perfectionistic features in childhood; and elevated scores tend to persist after symptomatic recovery.[5,7–9,37,49]

Recent research has extended the study of perfectionism to examine questions about causation, moderation, and mediation using longitudinal and experimental methods. Prospective research with an undergraduate sample determined that maladaptive perfectionism interacted with relationship- and appearance-contingent self-esteem to predict increased rates of disordered eating 14 months later.[48] In an experimental design with a nonclinical sample, an induction of the personal standards dimension of perfectionism was associated with increased weight concerns and bulimic symptoms for a subgroup of participants with elevated body dissatisfaction.[50] Both of these findings suggest that perfectionism may interact with other risk factors to precipitate ED symptomatology, at least in normal controls. In addition, it may be worthwhile to consider perfectionism within the broader context of self-evaluation and beliefs about self-worth. For example, patients with EDs have been shown to differ from a depressed clinical sample in reporting harsher self-criticism, in attributing their critical self-evaluation to their personalities, and in judging self-reproach to be more beneficial.[51]

Perfectionism is by no means uniquely associated with EDs, as it has been linked to depression, social anxiety, obsessive compulsive disorder, and OCPD as well as dysfunctional behaviors such as procrastination and burnout.[52,53] The relationship between perfectionism and EDs is distinctive, however, in both magnitude and pattern. Patients with AN in particular obtain astronomical scores, in one study yielding perhaps the highest group mean ever recorded for any sample on a widely used measure.[38,54]

Most notably, both positive and negative subscales are characteristically elevated, suggesting that the dimensions of achievement striving and evaluative concern may be jointly implicated in EDs.[37,48] This pattern has implications for refining the construct of perfectionism, highlighting the need to consider the domain in which a "relentless pursuit of excellence" is invested. It also illuminates some of the most unusual features of AN psychopathology relative to other psychiatric disorders and foreshadows the problem of resistance to change. Patients often cast their eating and weight control efforts as essential elements of a quest for self-improvement and consider both their ED symptoms and perfectionistic style consonant with valued objectives. In this context, even the harsh self-criticism associated with the darker side of perfectionism may be cultivated as an effective, if painful, tactic in support of a superordinate goal. The belief that self-castigation is functional may typify negative perfectionism more generally[55]; however, this conviction may be both more emphatic in individuals with ED than other clinical patients[51] and more accurate. Indeed, one of the most interesting aspects of the relationship between personality variables and EDs is that certain "maladaptive patterns of internal experience and behavior" are very nearly job requirements for practicing self-starvation in the midst of plenty.[56] In that sense, perfectionism and obsessionality can be construed not only as vulnerability factors but also as ability factors for extreme, sustained restriction.[16]

Impulsivity

Like perfectionism, impulsivity is a multifaceted construct that summarizes a variety of traits and behavior patterns, including the disposition to act on emotion, failure to anticipate consequences, difficulty persisting in tasks, intolerance for boredom, and desire for new stimuli and excitement.[57] Although much remains to be clarified about the differential importance of these features and the ways they interact, basic conceptual issues have been less contentious in this area. Traditional models of assessment characterize impulsivity as a relatively stable personality trait that can be assessed through self-report; however, there has been increasing emphasis on laboratory-based behavioral tasks and ecological momentary assessment to capture shifts in intraindividual impulsivity in the natural environment.[58]

Four key components of impulsivity have been identified through factor analysis: urgency, lack of planning, low perseverance, and sensation seeking.[15,57] Negative urgency, defined as the tendency to act rashly in response to distressing emotions, has emerged as the most consistent predictor of bulimic behaviors[57,59]; paralleling patterns on the temperamental trait of Novelty Seeking, sensation seeking is also elevated in binge-eating subgroups.[6,8,60]

Descriptive and meta-analytic reviews conclude that negative urgency is a risk factor for the onset of binge eating and predicts increases in the frequency of bulimic symptoms.[7,8,57,59] Scores on this index differentiate individuals with BN from normal control and AN samples. Patients with ANBP also score higher on negative urgency than those with ANR; however, some evidence suggests that purging rather than binge eating may be more strongly associated with impulsivity in an ANBP sample.[61] Associations to binge eating in BED are equivocal, as both patients with BED and non-binging overweight patients presenting to a weight loss clinic obtained comparably high scores on negative urgency.[62]

When binge eating occurs in the context of severe dietary restriction, as in ANBP and often BN, it can be interpreted as a fundamentally normal response to deprivation rather than a marker of pervasive problems with impulse control.[17,63] For a subgroup of patients, however, a predisposition to impulsive action across domains may play an important role in the development and maintenance of EDs. Impulsivity is an established transdiagnostic risk factor for a number of disordered behaviors, including substance abuse, gambling, nonsuicidal self-injury, and borderline personality disorder.[64,65] Individuals who are predisposed to take immediate action when distressed, to seek rewarding sensations, and to suspend their awareness of consequences are temperamentally ill-suited to the dreary routines of long-haul restriction. When attempting to suppress eating and weight, they are likely to develop patterns dominated by recurrent binge eating and purging behavior, whereas those with a stronger loading for perseverance and constraint are better matched to the rhythms and rituals of dieting.[66–68]

Impulsivity and compulsivity are often conceptualized as opposite ends of a spectrum; however, recent research suggests that the relationship between them is complex.[69,70] Although impulsivity predicts binge eating in patients with ED and compulsivity is most closely associated with restriction, these patterns can coexist, interact, and contribute jointly to the maintenance of disordered eating, with individuals high in both manifesting the most severe ED pathology.[71] A model proposed by Pearson, Wonderlich, and Smith[59] suggests that binge-purge behavior that is initially impulsive in nature acquires compulsive qualities as the pattern becomes entrenched, paralleling processes involved in the drug abuse model.

ALTERNATIVE PATHS AND PERSPECTIVES

After decades of research on personality dimensions and disorders in the ED field, the principal conclusions of an early review still apply.[5] When weight status and binge-purge behavior are used to sort cases into diagnostic categories, robust but imperfect associations are found between ED subtypes and traits. When personality patterns are examined within diagnoses, however, many patients do not match the temperamental profile of the category to which they belong. As long as symptom-based diagnostic groups are the focus of study, heterogeneity within categories and frequent crossover between them can obscure the role of temperamental factors in the initiation, course, and resolution of EDs.

In recent years, many investigators have chosen an alternative research strategy, sorting ED patients according to empirically derived personality prototypes rather than current symptom pattern. In one influential study, Westen and Harnden-Fischer[68] asked 103 psychiatrists and psychologists to characterize a patient with ED in their caseloads using descriptive items from a measure of personality pathology; Q-analysis was then conducted to reveal natural groupings. Two-thirds of cases could be allocated to one of the three types identified: a high-functioning subset and two groups manifesting substantial and divergent personality pathology. These prototypes predicted a range of phenomena better than ED diagnoses, including abuse history, previous hospitalization, and current functioning as well as unique variance in ED symptom patterns.[68]

Related approaches have yielded strikingly similar findings across varied ED samples, data sources, instruments, and analytical techniques.[8,11,66,72–76] Almost all replicate the three-group pattern, which has also emerged in research with other psychiatric patients and the general population. In ED samples, the following patterns recur:

Minimal Personality Pathology (Also Termed Low Psychopathology, High-Functioning, Normative, or Resilient)

A substantial minority show no signs of significant psychological disturbance other than the presenting symptoms, although they tend to be worried and perfectionistic relative to healthy controls. In mixed ED samples, subgroups of both patients with AN and patients with BN fit this profile, sometimes with an overrepresentation of BN. In one study that included clinical and recruited participants with full-syndrome or subthreshold BN, the low comorbidity cluster was the most common pattern identified.[77] Although the proportion of high-functioning individuals varies across samples and settings, the consistent emergence of this subtype provides an important reminder that not all patients are deeply disturbed, with the notable exception of the ED symptoms from which they currently suffer.

Overcontrolled/Constricted

This class is characterized by more pronounced and pervasive rigidity, inhibition, avoidance, dysphoria, and anhedonia, with high scores on Neuroticism and low levels of Extraversion. The dominant diagnoses are ANR and ANB, frequently comorbid with cluster C and sometimes schizoid personality disorders.

Undercontrolled/Emotionally Dysregulated

The most severe personality pathology is evident in the undercontrolled group, depicted as impulsive, affectively unstable, and oppositional. Binge eating is strongly associated with this subtype; in one study, 100% of patients in the undercontrolled group carried BN or ANB diagnoses, and none had an ANR history.[68] Patients who fit this group have more severe ED symptoms, greater comorbidity with cluster B personality disorders, higher rates of self-injury and substance use, more frequent hospitalizations, and poorer treatment outcomes.

Subtype analysis does not overcome all the limitations of diagnosis-bound personality assessment; for example, state and trait effects remain entangled in the profiles that emerge from cross-sectional data and little is known about subtype stability when assessed in acutely ill patients. In addition, because subtypes are generated for specific samples, the method does not yield standard scores or criteria that can be applied to other ED groups or individuals. Within studies, a varied proportion of cases cannot be classified into any of the clusters delineated, suggesting that the overcontrolled, undercontrolled, and low-psychopathology prototypes are not characteristic of all patients with ED.

Nonetheless, the shift in perspective afforded by this approach has multiple advantages. Rather than studying separate dimensions of personality in isolation, the method takes account of how traits work together.[78] For example, high levels of perfectionism may have different determinants and consequences if they are paired with a predisposition for impulsivity as opposed to paired with a pull toward constraint, yet these interactions may not be considered if the variables are examined independently.[79] Research on clusters of traits also helps to clarify the robust but puzzling finding of marked heterogeneity within diagnostic categories.[8,68] Such heterogeneity is not random but patterned, representing several distinct subsets of patients who differ on key personality dimensions. If data from high-functioning, perfectionistic patients with BN are combined with data from severely disturbed, undercontrolled patients with BN, this systematic within-group variability is cancelled out.[68,74] By contrast, a constricted, avoidant patient with BN may have more core features in common with a patient who has a similar personality profile than with a high-functioning or undercontrolled patient with BN with a matching diagnosis.[5,72]

Subtyping research may prove most generative to the extent that it refocuses attention on a recurrent theme in the ED literature: different temperamental characteristics may predispose individuals to develop EDs through different pathways, affecting not only the likelihood that eating/weight symptoms will emerge but the form they take, the functional relationships that maintain them, and the course they follow. Varied personality profiles also show differential patterns of association with genetic and environmental risk factors; for example, individuals in the low-psychopathology subgroup are more likely to have family members with EDs, while those with undercontrolled profiles report higher rates of childhood abuse.[68,69,72,80]

The idea that dissimilar individuals may be vulnerable to EDs for disparate reasons has been advanced in numerous models of AN[3,4,81] and BN,[77,82–84] while the subtyping approach provides a framework for examining these associations across diagnostic categories as well as within them. Instead of viewing the heterogeneity of personality features as unwelcome variance that obscures the identification of trait-symptom relationships, this perspective suggests that subgroup and individual differences in the determinants and functions of EDs should be sought and studied in their own right[5] and thoughtfully considered in the design of treatment approaches matched to the strengths and vulnerabilities represented in each constellation of traits.[72,73,75] For example, individuals who fit the overcontrolled profile may be especially reluctant to give up dietary restriction because it requires and rewards the very characteristics that define this subtype: constriction, Persistence, attention to detail, and the disposition to suppress or defer hedonic impulses.[73,85] These patients may benefit from treatments designed to enhance cognitive flexibility[72,86]; at the same time, their ability to make use of top-down regulation strategies can become an asset in the process of treatment.[75] Similarly, perfectionism can be viewed as both a target and a tool of change efforts for low-psychopathology patients who construe their ED symptoms as part of a self-improvement campaign. The drive to excel in a valued domain can be a powerful attribute when redirected to serve recovery.[6,87] Simultaneously, the harsh self-criticism that accompanies perfectionistic striving in these patients may be addressed through the use of self-compassion techniques as an adjunctive treatment component.[88,89]

Research on the link between personality patterns and alternative paths to EDs will be most instructive to the extent that it includes multiple modes of assessment and considers multiple levels of analysis in conjunction. For example, the subtyping approach can be combined with ecological momentary assessment to yield new insights about how personality profiles influence affect and behavior in the natural environment[76] and integrated with experimental and neurocognitive investigations to advance our understanding of underlying mechanisms.[72]

REFERENCES

1. Dubois FS. Compulsion neurosis with cachexia (anorexia nervosa). Am J Psychiatry 1949;106(2):107–15.
2. Widiger TA. Personality and psychopathology. World Psychiatry 2011;10(2): 103–6.
3. Dally P. Anorexia nervosa. New York: Grune & Stratton; 1973.
4. Strober M. An empirically derived typology of anorexia nervosa. In: Darby PL, Garner DM, Coscina DV, editors. Anorexia nervosa: recent developments in research. New York: Alan R. Liss; 1983. p. 185–96.
5. Vitousek KM, Manke FP. Personality variables and disorders in anorexia nervosa and bulimia nervosa. J Abnorm Psychol 1994;103(1):137–47.
6. Atiye M, Miettunen J, Raevuori-Helkamaaa A. A meta-analysis of temperament in eating disorders. Eur Eat Disord Rev 2015;23(2):89–99.
7. Cassin SE, von Ranson KM. Personality and eating disorders: a decade in review. Clin Psychol Rev 2005;25(7):895–916.
8. Farstad SM, McGeown LM, von Ranson KM. Eating disorders and personality, 2004-2016: a systematic review and meta-analysis. Clin Psychol Rev 2016;46: 91–105.
9. Lilenfeld LRR, Wonderlich S, Riso LP, et al. Eating disorders and personality: a methodological and empirical review. Clin Psychol Rev 2006;26(3):299–320.
10. Martinussen M, Friborg O, Schmierer P, et al. The comorbidity of personality disorders in eating disorders: a meta-analysis. Eat Weight Disord 2017;22(2):201–9.
11. Von Ranson KM. Personality and eating disorders. In: Wonderlich S, Mitchell JE, de Zwaan M, et al, editors. Annual review of eating disorders part 2. Oxford (UK): CRC Press; 2008. p. 84–96.
12. Wonderlich S, Mitchell JE. The role of personality in the onset of eating disorders and treatment implications. Psychiatr Clin North Am 2001;24(2):249–58.
13. Clark LA, Livesley J, Morey L. Personality assessment: the challenge of construct validity. J Pers Disord 1997;11(3):205–31.
14. Grilo CM, McGlashan TH, Oldham JM. Course and stability of personality disorders. J Psychiatr Pract 1998;4(2):61–75.
15. Whiteside SP, Lynam DR. The Five Factor Model and impulsivity: using a structural model of personality to understand impulsivity. Pers Individ Dif 2001;30(4): 669–89.

16. Vitousek KM, Stumpf RE. Difficulties in the assessment of personality traits and disorders in eating-disordered individuals. Eat Disord 2005;13(1):37–60.
17. Keys A, Brozek J, Henschel A, et al. The biology of human starvation. Minneapolis (MN): University of Minnesota Press; 1950.
18. Vitousek KM, Manke FP, Gray JA, et al. Caloric restriction for longevity: II—The systematic neglect of behavioural and psychological outcomes in animal research. Eur Eat Disord Rev 2004;12(6):338–60.
19. Anderluh M, Tchanturia k, Rabe-Hesketh S, et al. Lifetime course of eating disorders: design and validity testing of a new strategy to define the eating disorders phenotype. Psychol Med 2008;39:105–14.
20. Peat C, Mitchell JE, Hoek HW, et al. Validity and utility of subtyping anorexia nervosa. Int J Eat Disord 2009;42(7):590–4.
21. Tozzi F, Thornton LM, Klump KL, et al. Symptom fluctuation in eating disorders: correlates of diagnostic crossover. Am J Psychiatry 2005;162(4):732–40.
22. Fairburn CG, Cooper Z, Shafran R. Cognitive behavior therapy for eating disorders: a "transdiagnostic" theory and treatment. Behav Res Ther 2003;41(5): 509–28.
23. Rothbart MK, Ahadi SA, Evans DE. Temperament and personality: origins and outcomes. J Pers Soc Psychol 2000;78(1):122–35.
24. Cloninger CR. A systematic method for clinical description and classification of personality variants. Arch Gen Psychiatry 1987;44(6):573–88.
25. Digman JM. Personality structure: emergence of the Five-Factor Model. Annu Rev Psychol 1990;41(1):417–40.
26. Miettunen J, Raevuori A. A meta-analysis of temperament in axis I psychiatric disorders. Compr Psychiatry 2012;53(2):152–66.
27. Anderluh MB, Tchanturia K, Rabe-Hesketh S, et al. Childhood obsessive-compulsive personality traits in adult women with eating disorders: defining a broader eating disorder phenotype. Am J Psychiatry 2003;160(2):242–7.
28. Bulik CM, Hebebrand J, Keski-Rahkonen A, et al. Genetic epidemiology, endophenotypes, and eating disorder classification. Int J Eat Disord 2007;40:S52–60.
29. Råstam M. Anorexia nervosa in 51 Swedish adolescents: premorbid problems and comorbidity. J Am Acad Child Adolesc Psychiatry 1992;31(5):819–29.
30. Klump KL, Strober M, Bulik CM, et al. Personality characteristics of women before and after recovery from an eating disorder. Psychol Med 2004;34(8):1407–18.
31. Wagner A, Barbarich-Marsteller NC, Frank GK, et al. Personality traits after recovery from eating disorders: do subtypes differ? Int J Eat Disord 2006;39(4):276–84.
32. Strober M. Disorders of the self in anorexia nervosa: an organismic-developmental paradigm. In: Johnson C, editor. Psychodynamic treatment of anorexia nervosa and bulimia nervosa. New York: Guilford Press; 1992. p. 354–73.
33. Rowe S, Jordan J, McIntosh V. Dimensional measures of personality as a predictor of outcome at 5-year follow-up in women with bulimia nervosa. Psychiatry Res 2011;185(2):414–20.
34. Grilo CM. Recent research of relationships among eating disorders and personality disorders. Curr Psychiatry Rep 2002;4(1):18–24.
35. Sansone RA, Levitt JL, Sansone LA. The prevalence of personality disorders among those with eating disorders. Eat Disord 2005;13(1):7–21.
36. Stice E. Risk and maintenance factors for eating pathology: a meta-analytic review. Psychol Bull 2002;128(5):825–48.
37. Bardone-Cone AM, Wonderlich SA, Frost RO, et al. Perfectionism and eating disorders: current status and future directions. Clin Psychol Rev 2007;27(3): 384–405.

38. Flett GL, Hewitt PL. Measures of perfectionism. In: Boyle GJ, Saklofske DH, Matthews G, editors. Measures of personality and social psychological constructs. London (UK): Academic Press; 2015. p. 595–618.
39. Shafran R, Cooper Z, Fairburn CG. Clinical perfectionism: a cognitive-behavioural analysis. Behav Res Ther 2002;40(7):773–91.
40. Stairs AM, Smith GT, Zapolski TC, et al. Clarifying the construct of perfectionism. Assessment 2012;19(2):146–66.
41. Chin D. Defining perfectionism: popular and clinical conceptions. [master's thesis]. Honolulu (HI): University of Hawaiʻi at Mānoa; 1988.
42. Garner DM, Olmstead MP, Polivy J. Development and validation of a multidimensional eating disorder inventory for anorexia nervosa and bulimia. Int J Eat Disord 1983;2(2):15–34.
43. Frost RO, Marten P, Lahart C, et al. The dimensions of perfectionism. Cognit Ther Res 1990;14(5):449–68.
44. Hewitt PL, Flett GL. Perfectionism in the self and social contexts: conceptualization, assessment, and association with psychopathology. J Pers Soc Psychol 1991;60(3):456.
45. Flett GL, Hewitt PL. Positive versus negative perfectionism in psychopathology: a comment on Slade and Owens's dual process model. Behav Modif 2006;30(4):472–95.
46. Egan S, Piek J, Dyck M, et al. The reliability and valifity of the positive and negative perfectionism scale. Clin Psychol 2011;15(3):121–32.
47. Smith MM, Sherry SB, Chen S, et al. The perniciousness of perfectionism: a meta-analytic review of the perfectionism-suicide relationship. J Pers 2018;86(3):522–42.
48. Bardone-Cone AM, Lin SL, Butler RM. Perfectionism and contingent self-worth in relation to disordered eating and anxiety. Behav Ther 2017;48(3):380–90.
49. Culbert KM, Racine SE, Klump KL. Research review: what we have learned about the causes of eating disorders – A synthesis of sociocultural, psychological, and biological research. J Child Psychol Psychiatry 2015;56(11):1141–64.
50. Boone L, Soenens B. In double trouble for eating pathology? An experimental study on the combined role of perfectionism and body dissatisfaction. J Behav Ther Exp Psychiatry 2015;47:77–83.
51. Thew GR, Gregory JD, Roberts K, et al. The phenomenology of self-critical thinking in people with depression, eating disorders, and in healthy individuals. Psychol Psychother 2017;90(4):751–69.
52. Egan SJ, Wade TD, Shafran R. Perfectionism as a transdiagnostic process: a clinical review. Clin Psychol Rev 2011;31(2):203–12.
53. Hill AP, Curran T. Multidimensional perfectionism and burnout: a meta-analysis. Pers Soc Psychol Rev 2016;20(3):269–88.
54. Cockell SJ, Hewitt PL, Seal B, et al. Trait and self-presentational dimensions of perfectionism among women with anorexia nervosa. Cognit Ther Res 2002;26(6):745–58.
55. Egan SJ, Piek JP, Dyck M, et al. A clinical investigation of motivation to change standards and cognitions about failure in perfectionism. Behav Cogn Psychother 2013;41(5):565–78.
56. Vitousek KM, Gray JA, Grubbs KM. Caloric restriction for longevity: I. Paradigm, protocols, and physiological findings in animal research. Eur Eat Disord Rev 2004;12(5):279–99.

57. Fischer S, Smith GT, Cyders MA. Another look at impulsivity: a meta-analytic review comparing specific dispositions to rash action in their relationship to bulimic symptoms. Clin Psychol Rev 2008;28(8):1413–25.
58. Tomko RL, Solhan MB, Carpenter RW, et al. Measuring impulsivity in daily life: the momentary impulsivity scale. Psychol Assess 2014;26(2):339.
59. Pearson CM, Wonderlich SA, Smith GT. A risk and maintenance model for bulimia nervosa: from impulsive action to compulsive behavior. Psychol Rev 2015;122(3): 516–35.
60. Rosval L, Steiger H, Bruce K, et al. Impulsivity in women with eating disorders: problems of response inhibition, planning, or attention. Int J Eat Disord 2006; 39(7):590–3.
61. Hoffman ER, Gagne DA, Thornton LM, et al. Understanding the association of impulsivity, obsessions, and compulsions with binge eating and purging behaviours in anorexia nervosa. Eur Eat Disord Rev 2012;20(3):e129–36.
62. Nasser JA, Gluck ME, Geliebter A. Impulsivity and test meal intake in obese binge eating women. Appetite 2004;43(3):303–7.
63. Polivy J, Herman CP. Dieting and binging: a causal analysis. Am Psychol 1985; 40(2):193–201.
64. Reas DL, Pedersen G, Rø Ø. Impulsivity-related traits distinguish women with co-occurring bulimia nervosa in a psychiatric sample. Int J Eat Disord 2016;49: 1093–6.
65. Robbins TW, Gillan CM, Smith DG, et al. Neurocognitive endophenotypes of impulsivity and compulsivity: Towards dimensional psychiatry. Trends Cogn Sci 2012;16(1):81–91.
66. Keel P, Fichter M, Quadflieg N, et al. Application of a latent class analysis to empirically define eating disorder phenotypes. Arch Gen Psychiatry 2004;61: 192–200.
67. Klump KL, Bulik CM, Pollice C, et al. Temperament and character in women with anorexia nervosa. J Nerv Ment Dis 2000;188(9):559–67.
68. Westen D, Harnden-Fischer J. Personality profiles in eating disorders: rethinking the distinction between axis I and axis II. Am J Psychiatry 2001;158:547–62.
69. Wildes JE, Marcus MD. Incorporating dimensions into the classification of eating disorders: three models and their implications for research and clinical practice. Int J Eat Disord 2013;46(5):396–403.
70. Godier LR, Park RJ. Compulsivity in anorexia nervosa: a transdiagnostic concept. Front Psychol 2014;5:778.
71. Engel SG, Corneliussen SJ, Wonderlich SA. Impulsivity and compulsivity in bulimia nervosa. Int J Eat Disord 2005;38(3):244–51.
72. Wildes JE, Marcus MD. Alternative methods of classifying eating disorders: models incorporating comorbid psychopathology and associated features. Clin Psychol Rev 2013;33:383–94.
73. Wildes JE, Marcus MD, Crosby RD, et al. The clinical utility of personality subtypes in patients with anorexia nervosa. J Consult Clin Psychol 2011;79(5): 665–74.
74. Claes L, Vandereycken W, Luyten P, et al. Personality prototypes in eating disorders based on the Big Five model. J Pers Disord 2006;20(4):401–16.
75. Turner BJ, Claes L, Wilderjans TF, et al. Personality profiles in eating disorders: further evidence of the clinical utility of examining subtypes based on temperament. Psychiatry Res 2014;219:157–65.

76. Lavender JM, Wonderlich SA, Crosby RD, et al. Personality-based subtypes of anorexia nervosa: examining validity and utility using baseline clinical variables and ecological momentary assessment. Behav Res Ther 2013;51:512–7.
77. Wonderlich SA, Crosby RD, Joiner T, et al. Personality subtyping and bulimia nervosa: psychopathological and genetic correlates. Psychol Med 2005;35: 649–57.
78. Donnellan MB, Robbins RW. Resilient, overcontrolled, and undercontrolled personality types: issues and controversies. Soc Personal Psychol Compass 2010; 3:1–14.
79. Slof-Op't Landt MCT, Claes L, van Furth EF. Classifying eating disorders based on 'healthy' and 'unhealthy' perfectionism and impulsivity. Int J Eat Disord 2016;49: 673–80.
80. Holliday J, Landau S, Collier D, et al. Do illness characteristics and familial risk differ between women with anorexia nervosa grouped on the basis of personality pathology. Psychol Med 2006;36:529–38.
81. Sohlberg S, Strober M. Personality in anorexia nervosa: an update and a theoretical integration. Acta Psychiatr Scand 1994;89:1–15.
82. Steiger H, Bruce KR. Phenotypes, endophenotypes, and genotypes in bulimia spectrum eating disorders. Can J Psychiatry 2007;52:220–7.
83. Stice E. A prospective test of the dual-pathway model of bulimic pathology: mediating effects of dieting and negative affect. J Abnorm Psychol 2001;110(1): 124–35.
84. Lacey JH. Moderation of bulimia. J Psychosom Res 1984;28:397–402.
85. Vitousek K, Hollon S. The investigation of schematic content and processing in eating disorders. Cognit Ther Res 1990;14:191–214.
86. Tchanturia K, Lloyd S, Lang K. Cognitive remediation therapy for anorexia nervosa: current evidence and future research directions. Int J Eat Disord 2013;46: 492–5.
87. Vitousek K, Watson S, Wilson GT. Enhancing motivation for change in treatment-resistant eating disorders. Clin Psychol Rev 1998;18:391–420.
88. Gilbert P. Compassion focused therapy: distinctive features. New York: Routledge; 2010.
89. Gale C, Gilbert P, Read N, et al. An evaluation of the impact of introducing compassion-focused therapy to a standard treatment programme for people with eating disorders. Clin Psychol Psychother 2014;21(1):1–12.

The Role of Sociocultural Factors in the Etiology of Eating Disorders

Ruth Striegel Weissman, PhD

KEYWORDS

- Eating disorder • Etiology • Sociocultural factors • Risk factors • Culture
- Epidemiology • Acculturation • Ethnicity

KEY POINTS

- In the eating disorder field, the risk factor literature reflects a lack of methodological consistency, making it difficult to draw straightforward conclusions.
- The use of population-based registers and record linking is a major advance in the field because it allows for accumulating very large case samples and accessing high-quality risk factor data.
- Combining eating diagnoses into a transdiagnostic eating disorder category is premature.

INTRODUCTION

The individual does not exist apart from cultural influence, but is born into—and can only develop within—particular worlds that come culturally configured.
—Adams and Markus, 2004, p. 346.[1]

Research into risk factors for the development of any disorder is undertaken in hopes of improving understanding of and finding information needed for reducing the burden of suffering related to the disorder. Eating disorders (EDs) are associated with substantial personal and societal burdens, including alarmingly high mortality, extensive medical and psychiatric comorbidity, and substantial direct and indirect economic costs due to elevated health services utilization or adverse impacts on educational attainment or employment.[2–4] Hence, there is an urgency to answer the questions of who develops an ED, why, and under what circumstances. Risk factor studies may inform prevention interventions to eliminate or weaken the effect of modifiable risk factors (eg, exposure to media images of extremely thin fashion models) or, if the risk factor is not modifiable (eg, death of a parent), to provide support for at-risk

Disclosure Statement: Professor R.S. Weissman is Editor-in-Chief of the *International Journal of Eating Disorders* and receives a stipend for her role.
Department of Psychology, Wesleyan University, 207 High Street, Middletown, CT 06359, USA
E-mail address: rweissman@wesleyan.edu

individuals. Risk factor research also informs treatment development, as recently reviewed by Pennesi and Wade.[5]

The overrepresentation of girls and women among individuals with an ED,[6] the emergence of EDs at distinct historical periods and in geopolitically distinct regions of the world,[7,8] and the increased risk observed among individuals exposed through migration or the diffusion of ideas, images and values associated with cultures of modernity[9,10] have led scholars to theorize that sociocultural factors play an integral role in ED etiology.[5] In the past century, anorexia nervosa (AN) and bulimia nervosa (BN) were considered culture-bound syndromes and cross-cultural comparisons were undertaken to test this assumption. Yet, although early studies found differences in the incidence or prevalence when comparing samples representing Western culture or cultures of modernity with samples representing other cultures, recent reviews concluded that, increasingly, EDs are being identified in diverse countries and cultures worldwide.[8,11,12] A variant of testing the Western culture theory involves comparisons of subcultures within a country (eg, racial or ethnic minorities vs majority populations, or sexual minority vs sexual majority groups) with the guiding assumption that if these subcultures espouse different beauty ideals or differ on other cultural variables from the majority group, correspondingly, the minority groups should be less likely (or in the case of homosexual men, more likely) to experience EDs. Cultural developments, such as globalization and proliferation of social media, have contributed to broad dissemination of Western culture and, increasingly, research has found that individuals living in non-Western cultures or representing ethnic or sexual minority groups also are at risk for developing an ED.[8,13,14] Moreover, within a given culture, minority populations are not insulated from exposure to the majority culture's norms, institutions, or policies; rather, they are exposed to multiple and often conflicting cultural norms. Some studies suggest that such dual exposure may offset whatever protection a person might experience as a minority group member or even increase risk due to stresses arising from minority status (eg, discrimination).[15]

Early theoretic models focused on Western cultures' adoption of an unrealistically thin beauty ideal, norms of femininity that emphasized physical appearance as central to self-worth and interpersonal success, and gender-role proscriptions that limited girls' and women's agency and control over their lives.[16] The list of sociocultural risk factors has been greatly expanded, now encompassing culturally mediated processes, such as urbanization, transnational migration or acculturation, social environments (eg, sororities and sports teams) that might amplify certain harmful norms or values, and institutions or industries (media and agricultural or food conglomerates) responsible for the amplification or dissemination of risk factors.[2,9,17,18] This article reviews the recent (2016–2018) empirical literature describing studies on the contribution of sociocultural factors in ED etiology. Introduced first are challenges in studying ED etiology, followed by a description of how studies were selected for inclusion. Results then are summarized and a final section draws conclusions.

Key Challenges in Eating Disorders Risk Factor Research

Three challenges bear acknowledging:

1. Establishing precedence
2. What defines *sociocultural* risk factors is far from clear
3. Definitions of *dependent variables* vary greatly across studies

How these challenges informed the present article is discussed.

The term risk factor implies precedence
As Kraemer and colleagues noted,[18] a risk factor is "a measurable characteristic of a subject in a specified population which precedes the outcome of interest and which can be shown to divide the population into two groups: a high- and a low-risk group."[18(p20)] "Fixed markers" are risk variables that precede onset and cannot be shown to be changed (eg, gender at birth). The requirement of temporal precedence limits the designs suitable for testing risk factor hypotheses. Although fixed markers can be established using cross-sectional designs, identifying modifiable risk factors requires longitudinal or experimental designs.[19] Increasingly, investigators have used hybrid designs involving linking of population-based registers for extracting risk factor data that had been collected in real time well prior to ED onset.

This review reports on results referring to variables where exposure occurred prior to ED onset and excludes studies examining risk for symptom maintenance or worsening.[20] Although correlations with unknown temporal sequence are useful for generating risk hypotheses, such correlate findings were not considered.

Lack of a common list of sociocultural risk factors
Many ED theories acknowledge culture as an important risk domain, yet what social variables beyond gender or race/ethnicity or what cultural factors beyond the ubiquitously noted "thin female beauty ideal" should be studied is far from clear. The first comprehensive review identified some 40 potential ED risk factors and classified 4 as "general and social factors": gender, race/ethnicity, participation in weight-related social or professional subculture, and sexual orientation.[18] The universe of sociocultural factors can be delineated by focusing on cultural theories of EDs; yet, a systematic review of ED theories identified more than 50 theoretic models, each enumerating multiple ED risk factors. Most theories implicate some cultural or social factors. Some risk factors are model-specific, whereas many others (eg, female gender, thin-ideal internalization, low self-esteem, and adverse interpersonal experiences) are named in multiple theories or, although referenced as model-specific, are conceptually similar to other variables (eg, appearance anxiety, body shame, and fear of weight gain).[5]

The most widely studied cultural theory of ED is objectification theory.[21–23] It posits that cultures where the female body is objectified (seen as a tool for the sexual pleasure and gratification of men) put girls or women at increased ED risk through mediating mechanisms, such as self-objectification, thin-ideal internalization, body shame, or body surveillance. A meta-analysis of 53 cross-sectional studies found moderately strong positive statistical associations between self-objectification and disordered eating.[21] Longitudinal studies are now needed for testing body objectification (a cultural norm or gender-role proscription) or self-objectification (as the internalization of the cultural norm) as an ED risk factor.

Another approach to testing cultural theories involves comparing individuals who have undergone a cultural transition via temporary[10] or permanent migration[24] or due to political or economic changes.[25] Often the focus is on whether cultural transition is associated with increases in ED prevalence rather than on any sociocultural factor that might explain ED risk.

ED risk is multifactorial both within a domain (here sociocultural factors) and across other major risk domains.[2] Consistent with Adams and Markus,[1] cultural influences cannot be cleanly separated from other risk domains. Yet, few studies have investigated multiple risk factors across major risk domains or used analytic strategies suitable for examining how risk factors might work together to result in distinct vulnerability pathways and corresponding risk groups.[26] Adding yet further complexity, ED risk factors cover a broad developmental spectrum (ranging from prenatal exposure to experiences into adolescence and possibly adulthood) and a given risk factor may not apply uniformly across all ages but rather may be developmentally specific.[2,18,27,28]

Given the lack of a commonly agreed-on set of sociocultural variables, this review follows the recommendation[18] to take an atheoretic approach and identified studies for review using an inclusive search term ("risk factor") and search terms associated with major methodological approaches to identifying sociocultural risk factors (eg, "acculturation").

Risk for what outcome?

Risk factor studies have used various approaches to defining the dependent variable:

1. Using ED diagnoses, with AN and BN the most commonly studied[28]
2. Transdiagnostically combining diagnoses into one ED category, with the stated rationale that transition from one to another ED diagnosis is common and that all EDs share common risk factors
3. Targeting an ED symptom (eg, body image disturbance or binge eating)
4. Creating a disordered eating variable

The question of whether EDs should be combined into one transdiagnostic category has not yet been settled. For example, both the likelihood of diagnostic transitions and of transition patterns vary across ED diagnoses (eg, lifetime comorbidity among EDs is lowest for AN and highest for binge-eating disorder [BED]; transition from AN to BED is far less common than from AN to BN).[29–33] Furthermore, diagnostic transition patterns have been shown to predict clinical course, which, along with risk factor findings, has been used as a criterion for diagnostic validity.[34] Studies using a transdiagnostic case definition may miss risk effects if a given variable increases risk for one but not another ED. Symptom-based outcomes have the advantage over syndrome-based approaches of increased case samples; for example, far more individuals report binge eating than meet diagnostic criteria for BN or BED.[32,33,35] Symptom-based outcomes have been widely used, including in prevention trials,[15,28,36,37] yet few individuals with an ED symptom ultimately develop an ED. The lack of a widely accepted composite "disordered eating" category complicates study comparisons; moreover, composite scores have the same limitations as transdiagnostic ED categories due to the heterogeneity of symptoms grouped into one score.[38] This review describes studies focusing on either ED diagnoses or a transdiagnostic ED category and excludes studies or findings regarding symptom-based outcomes.

Method

A PubMed search was conducted for journal articles published in English between January 1, 2016, and July 15, 2018, using the following terms: [sociocultural OR cultural OR cross-cultural OR culture OR acculturation OR acculturative OR risk factor(s) OR etiology OR etiologic OR epidemiology OR epidemiological] AND [anorexia nervosa OR bulimia nervosa OR binge-eating disorder OR purging disorder OR ARFID OR eating disorder(s)]. The search yielded 302 citations. Each article's abstract was reviewed considering the aforementioned inclusion/exclusion criteria. Additionally, articles were discarded if they did not report data (eg, reviews and study protocols); discussed but did not study risk factors; focused solely on a risk domain other than culture (eg, genetic studies); examined cultural differences in symptom expression, treatment response, or health services use; or had fewer than 20 case samples. Twenty-two risk factor studies were retained and are discussed.

Update on Risk Factor Research in Eating Disorders

Overview

Most studies included individuals with AN (18 studies) or BN (18 studies); individuals with BED or PD were included in 9 and 6 studies, respectively; 1 study used a code capturing all EDs, and 1 study focused on feeding and eating disorders (FEDs) in infants; 11 studies excluded boys and men. ED onset age was reported in 4 studies and varied by diagnosis: earliest onsets were found for AN (median 16[39]; means: 17.40–19.30[31,40,41]), followed by BN (mean 20.20[31]; mean 21.22[41]) and highest onset ages reported for BED (mean 23.15[41]; mean 24.50)[31]; 16 studies reported information on incidence or prevalence; yet, given differences in sampling strategies, ED definitions and assessment methods, not surprisingly, incidence and prevalence estimates varied considerably. Novel contributions of these studies are the inclusion of purging disorder (PD), which was found quite common,[39,42,43] and of FED in very young children. In several studies,[32,39–41] lifetime or cumulative incidence estimates were higher than previously reported (partly reflecting the change in diagnostic criteria) and, in 2 studies prevalence of AN even exceeded that of BN.[31,32]

Demographic characteristics indicating sociocultural risk

By providing information about a disorder's distribution in the population, epidemiologic studies are a key resource for identifying fixed markers, which are commonly used as proxies for sociocultural factors, including gender, ancestry, and parental education or income. Findings from 13 studies are summarized in **Table 1**. Shown first are studies of nationally representative adult samples in Switzerland[41] and the United States,[31] followed by a multiethnic study in the United Kingdom, with participants ages 16 to 90.[42] Shown next are studies of adolescent or young adults in Germany,[32,43] Finland,[40] and Mexico,[44] followed by 2 studies focused on middle-aged women in England[39] and in Puerto Rico.[45] Shown last are 4 record linkage studies based on Danish and/or Swedish patient registry data.[24,46–48]

Gender

Where both genders were included, girls or women outnumber boys or men in all ED categories. Transdiagnostic groupings (any ED) obscure the fact that female-to-male ratios vary across diagnosis. For example, gender differences in incidence or prevalence are smallest for BED, raising the question of what sociocultural factors might explain differential risk relative to BN with which BED shares core symptoms with the notable exception of inappropriate compensatory behaviors. A growing literature supports adding weight/shape concerns (a defining symptom of BN) to the BED criteria. Hence, clinically, the key distinction between BN and BED arises from dietary restraint and inappropriate compensatory behaviors.[49] In the only study of FED, hazard ratios (HRs) for gender were highest for babies diagnosed in their first year and nonsignificant when FED was first diagnosed in the second or third year of life.[48]

Ancestry

Prior reviews have noted the need to move beyond studying individuals representing majority cultures in Europe, North America, and Australia or New Zealand. The studies included still are heavily skewed toward such samples. Methodological differences, including use of different indicators for prevalence or incidence across studies, preclude confident interpretation of the results concerning race/ethnicity or nationality as a risk factor. For example, a Mexican study[44] identified 40 ED incident cases over an 8-year period based on state-of-the-art methods, finding incidence estimates comparable to studies of non-Hispanic samples. Yet, the sample comprised emerging adults, the group at highest risk for ED onset. Typically, in adult samples, increasing

Table 1
Key methodological features and findings of studies of fixed markers for eating disorders

Citation	Study Location and Sample Characteristics	Eating Disorder Identification, Diagnostic Criteria, and Study Instruments	Incidence or Point Prevalence or Lifetime Prevalence (95% CI)	Fixed Markers	Comments
Mohler-Kuo et al,[41] 2016	Switzerland Nationally representative sample of 10,038 residents ages 15–60 y (52% female)	DMS-IV (and DSM-5 for AN) Two-stage sampling Stage 1 involved telephone calls using questions about "household structure." Stage 2: CIDI 3.0, by phone	Weighted lifetime prevalence Female Any ED: 5.3% (4.7–5.9) AN: 1.9% (1.6–2.3) BN: 2.4% (2.0–2.8) BED: 2.4% (2.0–2.8) Male Any ED: 1.5% (1.1–1.9) AN: 0.2% (0.1–0.4) BN: 0.9% (0.6–1.2) BED: 0.7% (0.5–1.0) Weighted 12-mo prevalence Female Any ED: 1.5% (1.1–1.8) AN: 0.07% (0.03–0.2) BN: 0.6% (0.2–0.8) BED: 0.9% (0.6–1.2) Male Any ED: 1.5% (1.1–1.9) AN: 0.03% (0.004–0.02) BN: 0.5% (0.3–0.7) BED: 0.3% (0.5–1.0)	Gender Female > male across all EDs; statistical comparisons are not reported Ancestry, parental education, or income Not reported	Onset age: across EDs, a majority of cases have onsets between 10 y and 20 y of age. Approximately 75% of AN, 13% and 20% for BN and BED, respectively, reported onset before age 20.

Udo & Grilo,[31] 2018	United States Nationally representative sample of 36,309 noninstitutionalized civilians ages 18 y or older 2012–2013 National Epidemiologic Survey Study on Alcohol and Related Conditions Mean ages (SE) of ED sample AN: 41.8 (0.96) y BN: 39.1 (2.45) y BED: 45.2 (1.21) y	DSM-5 Alcohol Abuse and Alcohol Use Disorder and Associated Disabilities Interview Schedule 5, in person	Weighted lifetime prevalence Female AN: 1.42% (SE 0.12) BN: 0.46% (SE 0.6) BED: 1.25% (SE 0.10) Male AN: 0.12% (SE 0.04) BN: 0.08% (SE 0.03) BED: 0.42% (SE 0.06) Weighted 12-mo prevalence Female AN: 0.08% (SE 0.03) BN: 0.22% (SE 0.05) BED: 0.60% (SE 0.07) Male AN: 0.01% (SE 0.01) BN: 0.05% (SE 0.02) BED: 0.26% (SE 0.05)	Shown are adjusted OR (95% CI) Gender AN: 12.00 (6.45–22.34) BN: 5.80 (2.82–11.92) BED: 3.01 (2.17–4.16) Ancestry for lifetime diagnosis (reference group: non-Hispanic white) Hispanic AN: 0.48 (0.33–0.72) BN: 0.65 (0.33–1.29) BED: 0.75 (0.38–0.92) Non-Hispanic black AN: 0.19 (0.11–0.33) BN: 0.54 (0.25–1.19) BED: 0.60 (0.38–0.92) Parental education or income not reported	Age of onset: significantly later in BED vs AN or BN Gender: for each ED, lifetime prevalence was significantly greater in women than men. Ancestry: lifetime prevalence of AN was significantly more common in non-Hispanic white individuals vs non-Hispanic black or Hispanic individuals; lifetime prevalence of BN did not vary significantly by race/ethnicity; there were significantly fewer non-Hispanic black individuals than non-Hispanic white individuals with BED, whereas prevalence of BED did not differ significantly between Hispanic and non-Hispanic white individuals.

(continued on next page)

Table 1
(continued)

Citation	Study Location and Sample Characteristics	Eating Disorder Identification, Diagnostic Criteria, and Study Instruments	Incidence or Point Prevalence or Lifetime Prevalence (95% CI)	Fixed Markers	Comments
Solmi et al,[42] 2016	United Kingdom Cross-sectional prevalence study South East London Community Health Study 1698 individuals ages 16–90 y (66% female- 25.4% minority) Study sample N = 145 Mean age of interview sample 36.4 y	DSM-5 Two-stage case and control selection Stage 1: SCOFF Stage 2: SCID in person, if SCOFF score ≥2 or, for controls, <2 and negative screen for psychiatric disorders	Weighted 12-mo prevalence Entire sample Any ED: 7.4% (4.1%–13.0%) AN: 0 cases Female Any ED: 6.7% (3.1%–13.6%) BN: 1.2% (0.5%–2.7%) BED: 4.7% (1.7%–12.5%) PD: 0.8% (0.3%–2.2%) OSFED: 3.4% (1.2%–9.3%) Male Any ED: 0.9% (0.2%–4.1%) BN: 0 BED: 0.9% (0.2%–4.2%) PD: 0 OSFED: 0	Gender No male cases of BN, PD, OSFED BED: female 9/109, male 2/30, NS Ancestry ED sample predominantly white, no details provided Parental education or income not reported	For establishing the interview sample, ED screen positive cases were matched to ED screen negative controls on gender. 54.9% of participants eligible for enrollment to be interviewed declined or were lost to follow-up. ED diagnoses were made 2–3 y after administration of the SCOFF and were based retrospectively for the 12 mo preceding the time when the SCOFF was administered. "Any ED" included "OSFED" Sample size may have been too small to detect differences in fixed markers.

Source	Country/Sample	DSM/Method	Results	Gender/Sociocultural	Conclusions
Nagl et al,[32] 2016	Germany Representative community sample of 3021[1] adolescents and young adults from metropolitan Munich, Germany, Early Developmental Stages of Psychopathology study Ages 14–24 at baseline and ages 21–34 y at 10-y follow-up	DSM-IV Munich CIDI 3.0	Age-specific, weighted cumulative incidence by age 33: Female AN: 3.24% (2.5%–4.3%) BN: 2.2% (1.6%–3.1%) Male AN: 0.2% (0.07%–0.6%) BN: 0.08% (0.01%–0.5%) Weighted baseline 12-mo prevalence Female AN: 0.4% (0.2%–0.9%) BN: 0.3% (0.2%–0.7%) Male No AN or BN cases	Gender (cumulative incident up to the age at last assessment) OR 22.5 (95% CI, 8.7–58.6) Ancestry, parental education, or income are not reported	Peak threshold incidence periods for AN and BN: 13–18 y Gender: cumulative incidence up to the age at last assessment of AN or BN was significantly higher in females than males.
Hammerle et al,[43] 2016	Germany 1654 German 7th-grade and 8th-grade students from 9 schools in the state of Rhineland-Palatinate. Mean age 13.4 (SD 0.8) y	DSM-5 Structured Interview for Anorexia and Bulimia Nervosa–Self Report, in person Objective measures of height/weight	Unweighted prevalence AN: 0.3% (0.1–0.7) BN: 0.8% (0.4–1.4) BED: 0.5% (0.2–0.9) OSFED: atypical AN: 3.6% (2.7–4.5)- PD: 1.9% (1.3–2.7)	Gender Female/male ratio AN: 5:0 BN: 5:1 BED: 5:3 Atypical AN: 45:13 PD: 22:9 Parental education, parental income, ancestry not reported	Gender difference reached statistical significance for atypical AN and PD but no other diagnosis

(continued on next page)

Table 1
(continued)

Citation	Study Location and Sample Characteristics	Eating Disorder Identification, Diagnostic Criteria, and Study Instruments	Incidence or Point Prevalence or Lifetime Prevalence (95% CI)	Fixed Markers	Comments
Mustelin et al,[40] 2016	Finland Wave 4 of the FinnTwin16 birth cohorts study Nationwide sample of twins born in 1975–1979, restricted to those pairs where at age 16, both twins were alive and resided in Finland; only women were included Sample size N = 2285 Age range 22–27 y Mean age 24.4 (SD 0.9) y	*DSM-5* Two-stage case finding Stage 1: EDI subscales, self-reported ED, being suspected by others to have an ED, current and past minimum weight Stage 2: *DSM-IV* SCID via telephone, if screen positive, if twin of a screen positive case, or if randomly selected from among screen-negative participants	15-y incidence (age interval 10–24 y) of AN: 230 per 100,000 cases (180–280) per person-year Lifetime prevalence (unweighted): AN: 3.6% (2.7%–4.2%)	None reported	Gender: study sample included only women

Benjet et al,[44] 2016	Mexico
	1074 young adults who had participated 8 y before in a study of adolescent residents of Mexico City metropolitan area.
	Age range 12–26 y
		DSM-IV
		CIDI 3.0, adolescent version at Wave 1, adult version at Wave 2, in person
			8-y incidence (covering ages 12–26 y):
			Any ED: 3.7%
			Female 4.3%
			Male 3.1%
			Female
			  AN: 0.9%
			  Bulimia: 2.7%
			  Binge eating: 1.7%
			Male
			  AN: 1.7%
			  Bulimia: 0.8%
			  Binge eating: 0.8%
				Gender
				ED relative risk ratio 1.33 female, NS
				Bulimia but not anorexia or binge eating incidence significantly greater in females than males.
				Ancestry
				Not reported
				Parental education, parental income
				Not living with both parents
				Each tested for "any ED," NS
					Published article uses terms, *anorexia, bulimia,* and *binge eating,* but it seems implied that these terms refer to full-syndrome EDs.
					Incidence case sample is very small (14 male and 26 female ED cases).
					Fixed markers as measured at Wave I

Micali et al,[39] 2017	United Kingdom 5658 women who were the main carers of a child enrolled in the UK Avon Longitudinal Study of Parents and Children Phase 2 sample N = 1036 Mean age 47.78 (SD 4.5) y	DSM-IV/DSM-5 Two-phase assessment Phase 1: EDDS questionnaire Phase 2: SCID for DSM-IV (Revised), in person, including screen positive cases and a similar number of screen-negative women	Weighted lifetime prevalence AN: 3.64 (2.81–4.72) BN: 2.15 (1.7–2.74) BED: 1.96 (1.52–2.51) PD: 1.28 (0.85–1.92) OSFED (including PD): 7.64 (6.32–9.24)	Gender DNA Ancestry, parental education, or income not reported	Gender: all-female sample
O'Brien et al,[45] 2017	United States Cross-sectional prevalence study Sister Study 47,759 US or Puerto Rico women Age range 35–74 y Mean age 55.8 (9.0) no ED; 49.8 (7.7) ED cases	DSM-5 (AN or BN; only cases with onset between ages 9 y and 22 y were included) ED diagnosis based on self-report (Have you ever had anorexia nervosa or bulimia?) Fixed marker information: retrospective questionnaire Markers based on was age 13	Unweighted prevalence of AN or BN with onset between 9 and 22 y): 2%	Gender DNA Results shown below are adjusted OR (95% CI). Ancestry (reference group non-Hispanic white) Non-Hispanic black: 0.29 (0.19, 0.42) Hispanic: 0.47 (0.33, 0.74) Other: 0.78 (0.52, 1.19) Parental education (reference group high school or less) Some college: 1.27 (1.06, 1.53) Bachelor's degree: 1.67 (1.41, 1.98) Graduate degree: 2.13 (1.78, 2.56) Income not reported Food insecurity Ever vs never: 1.30 (1.03, 1.63)	Gender: All female sample Ancestry: Non-Hispanic white > ED prevalence than Hispanic, non-Hispanic black, or Other, respectively Parental education: ED significantly more prevalent among offspring whose parents had some college, a bachelor's degree, or a graduate degree, respectively, compared with high school or less Food insecurity: women who reported that their family did not have enough to eat were significantly more likely to self-report AN or BN compared with women who had never experienced food insecurity before ED onset.

(continued on next page)

Table 1
(continued)

Citation	Study Location and Sample Characteristics	Eating Disorder Identification, Diagnostic Criteria, and Study Instruments	Incidence or Point Prevalence or Lifetime Prevalence (95% CI)	Fixed Markers	Comments
Hvelplund et al,[48] 2016	Denmark 901,227 children born from 1997 to 2010, alive and living in Denmark until age 48 mo	ICD-10 codes for FEDs All data were extracted from population and patient registries	Cumulative incidence 1365 children, 1.6 per 1000 live births	Gender Female/male ratio: 1.1:0.9 HR 1.20 (95% CI, 1.08–1.42) Ancestry (immigration status; reference group native born) Both parents HR 2.24 (1.92–2.61) One immigrant parent HR 1.30 (1.10–1.54) Parental education or income not reported	Gender: FEC is more common in girls than boys Ancestry: FED more common in children with one or both parents born outside of Denmark
Razaz & Cnattingius,[46] 2018	Sweden 488,688 singleton girls born in Sweden from 1992 to 2002 as per Patient Registry and Cause of Death Register linked with Education Register and the Total Population Register AN case sample (diagnosed by 2012) N = 2414 (0.5%)	ICD-9 code 307B and ICD-10 codes F500 or F501, based on nation-wide Patient Registry and Cause of Death Register Demographic information (maternal education and country of origin) extracted from the Education and the Total Population Registers	Overall incidence rate of 8.54 per 10,000 person-years	Gender DNA [2]Adjusted HR (95% CI) Ancestry (Reference group: mother born in a Nordic country) Mother born in a non-Nordic country: HR = 0.63 (95% CI 0.52–0.76) Maternal education (Reference group < 9 years of schooling) 10–11: HR = 1.20 (95% CI 0.97–1.48)	Gender: all female sample Ancestry: significantly lower risk for AN in females whose mothers had been born in a non-Nordic country Maternal education: incidence of AN in daughters increased significantly in a dose-response pattern with increasing levels of maternal education.

Study	Sample	Measure	Prevalence	Variables examined / Results	Findings
Sundquist et al,[47] 2017	Sweden 5,397,675 individuals ages 18 y or older as per Primary Care Register for 9 regions in Sweden (1998 2016), linked with Education Register. AN case sample N = 12,633	ICD-10 code F50 (includes AN, BN, BED, ARFID, other specified EDs, and unspecified EDs)	0.2% of all individuals who were at least once registered in the Primary Care Register	Gender. Gender ratio in prevalence female/male: 10.33 (9.70; 11.01). Ancestry Not reported. Mean parental education (average across 5 levels) OR: 1.11 (1.09; 1.13). Income not reported. 12: HR = 1.40 (95% CI 1.12-1.73); 13–14: HR =1.64 (95% CI 1.32-2.04); ≥15: HR = 1.90 (95% CI 1.54-2.35)	Gender: ED significantly more common in women vs men. Mean parental education: OR illustrates the decreased odds per 1 SD increase in education. Risk for ED increased significantly with increased level of parental education.
Mustelin et al,[24] 2017	Denmark 1,184,205 individuals born from 1984 to 2002, as per population registers. Sweden 1,222,593 individuals born from 1889 to 1999, as per population registers. Inclusion criteria: child was alive and the child and both parents were residing in Denmark or Sweden, respectively, on child's 10th birthday.	ICD-10. Patient registers (hospital and outpatient). Reported here: AN, BN. Foreign migration codes[1]: first-generation immigrant (person and both parents born abroad)[2]; second-generation immigrant by both foreign-born parents (person him/herself born in Denmark/Sweden)[3]; second-	EDs across immigration status. Denmark AN: 4650 females, 359 males. BN: 2355 females, approximately 55 males (numbers too low for exact reporting in some of the immigration status categories). Sweden	Analyses focused on immigration status only; reference group: offspring and parents are native born. Reported are IRR, 95% CI, adjusted for calendar year and age. Immigration status Females, AN, Denmark 1. IRR 0.40 (0.29-0.53) 2. IRR 0.42 (0.34-0.50) 3. IRR 1.18 (1.02-1.62) Females, AN, Sweden	Gender: females > males in both countries and for both AN and BN. Very small case sample of male immigrants with BN in Denmark and N = 0 in male immigrants in Swedish sample. Immigration status: male and female first-generation immigrants[1] are at significantly lower risk for AN and BN, both in Denmark and Sweden (continued on next page)

Table 1
(continued)

Citation	Study Location and Sample Characteristics	Eating Disorder Identification, Diagnostic Criteria, and Study Instruments	Incidence or Point Prevalence or Lifetime Prevalence (95% CI)	Fixed Markers	Comments
	Individuals were followed from their 10th birthday until ED onset, death, emigration from Denmark/Sweden, or end of the follow-up period (end of 2013, Denmark, 2009 Sweden), whichever occurred first.	generation immigrant by foreign-born mother[4]; second-generation immigrant by foreign-born father; reference group: native Dane/ Swede (person and parents born in Denmark or Sweden)	AN: 3424 females, 268 males BN: 648 females, 9 males	1. IRR 0.25 (0.19–0.32) 2. IRR 0.35 (0.45–0.62) Males, AN, Denmark 1. IRR 0.25 (0.04–0.78) 2. IRR 0.45 (0.21–0.82) Males, AN, Sweden 1. IRR 0.52 (0.284–0.98) Females, BN, Denmark 1. IRR 0.62 (0.43–0.85) 2. IRR 0.57 (0.43–0.73) 3. IRR 1.97 (1.67–2.31) Females, BN, Sweden 1. IRR 0.30 (0.18–0.52) 2. IRR 1.37 (1.01–1.87) 3. IRR 1.48 (1.13–1.96)	Second-generation immigrants with both foreign-born parents[2] are at lower risk for AN in the Danish sample and in the female (but not male) Swedish sample. In the female Danish sample, risk for AN was elevated in second-generation females with a foreign-born father.[4] In regard to BN, findings varied by country, gender, and immigration category. In females, both in the Danish and Swedish samples, lower risk was observed in first-generation Immigrants and higher risks were found in second-generation immigrants with foreign-born fathers.

Only findings regarding "any eating disorder," AN, BN, BED, PD, or Other Specified Eating Disorders (OSFED) are included.
Abbreviations: CIDI, Composite International Diagnostic Interview 3.0; *DSM-5, Diagnostic and Statistical Manual of Mental Disorders* (Fifth Edition); *ICD-9, International Classification of Diseases, Ninth Revision;* NS, not statistically significant; OR, odds ratio; SCID, Structured Clinical Interview for DSM.

age and age cohort are associated with decreasing incidence and prevalence esti-mates whereas in children, increasing age is associated with higher estimates.[41,45,50] Two studies examined differences between non-Hispanic white (white), non-Hispanic black (black) Hispanic individuals, yielding two overarching findings: (1) that EDs were least common in black individuals and most common in white participants[31,45] and (2) in the only study to test for differences by ED diagnosis, that the degree of differences by race/ethnicity varied across EDs (largest, and statistically significant, for AN and smallest for BED).[31] Udo and Grilo[31] cautioned that the prevalence estimates for BN and BED in the US study were unusually low in all ancestry groups; hence, the findings of no differences across racial/ethnic groups in the prevalence of BN await replication.

Parental socioeconomic status
In 3 of 4 studies that reported on indicators of parental socioeconomic status, higher levels of parental education were associated with increased risk for AN[46] or risk for ED.[45,47] The exception was 1 study where neither parental educational nor family in-come was associated significantly with ED risk, but the ED sample was small.[44] ED risk also was elevated in women who had experienced food insecurity (a proxy mea-sure of family poverty),[45] a result that is consistent with a recent study of elevated prevalence of ED symptoms in patrons of soup kitchens or food pantries.[51]

Immigration
Results from three studies with data on immigration status suggest that risk varied by ED. Specifically, FEC was more commonly diagnosed in children born to one or both immigrant parents versus children of parents born in Denmark,[48] but the early onset and the extensive biological risk factors associated with FED in infants suggest that FED is etiologically distinct from EDs with onsets in older children or adults.[52]

A second study reported significantly lower risk for AN in Swedish girls whose mothers had been born in a non-Nordic country.[46] A third study involving individuals born in Denmark or Sweden specifically focused on immigrants versus the reference group of native-born offspring of native-born parents.[24] ED risk was significantly lower in first-generation immigrants. Results concerning ED risk in second-generation immi-grant children varied by country, diagnosis, and gender of the child.[24] Among girls and women in both countries, risk for AN was significantly lower in second-generation im-migrants with two foreign-born parents; in sons, AN risk was lower only in the Danish. Moreover, risk for AN was elevated in second-generation daughters with a foreign-born father in the Danish sample only.

In regard to BN, male samples were too small for statistical tests. In Danish and Swedish girls and women, lower risk was observed in first-generation immigrants and higher risk in second-generation immigrants with foreign-born fathers. In the Danish but not Swedish sample, second-generation daughters with two foreign-born parents had lower risk for BN. Measured only in the Danish sample, foreign-born adoptees and daughters born to expatriates had higher risk for BN.

Lower prevalence among first-generation immigrants has been well documented for several psychiatric disorders, but as the investigators noted, the risk-lowering effect of immigrant status was especially strong in AN, where risk was nearly halved among first-generation immigrants or immigrants with two foreign-born parents. Because ED diagnoses were extracted from patient registers, difference across immigrant groups partly may reflect differences in treatment seeking or detection patterns. Prior research found that failure to seek treatment or be properly diagnosed when present-ing for treatment was more common among individuals with BED than AN or BN, mi-norities, and boys and men.[4] Future studies should explore why marriage involving a native-born and a foreign-born partner is associated with increased ED risk for offspring. For example, perhaps these couples experience higher levels of unresolved family disagreements, a variable reported to increase risk for AN or BN in two case-control studies.[53,54]

Studies exploring variable risk factors

Variable risk factor studies examined data across 3 prevention trials designed to reduce ED risk in at-risk women;[26] tested risk using classification tree analysis (CTA);[55,56] used a case-control design and retrospectively measured exposure to more than 120 risk factors;[53,54] or used register-based record linkage designs to test the role of early childhood adversities;[57–59] immigration status;[24] or school characteristics[60] in the etiology of EDs. Only findings pertaining to AN, BN, or BED are discussed.

Multidomain risk factor studies

Using data from 3 targeted prevention trials, including 1271 women (mean age 18.5; SD 4.2) with high levels of body image concerns (but not an ED diagnosis), Stice and colleagues[26] tested whether these baseline characteristics were predictive of ED onset: thin-ideal internalization, thinness expectancy (expecting positive outcomes from being thin), denial of thin-ideal costs, body dissatisfaction, dieting, negative affect, overeating, fasting, excessive exercise, functional impairment, mental health care, and body mass index (BMI). There were 9 women with AN, 77 with BN, 69 with BED, and 53 with PD. Multivariate models identified these significant predictors of ED onset: elevated negative affect (95% CI, HR 2.23; 1.25–3.99) and lower BMI (95% CI, HR 0.63; 0.44–0.91) for AN, body dissatisfaction (95% CI, HR 1.50; 1.08–2.08), overeating (95% CI, HR 2.07; 1.65–2.61), and fasting (95% CI, HR 1.29; 1.08–1.53) for BN, body dissatisfaction (95% CI, HR 1.49; 1.07–2.06), overeating (95% CI, HR 1.99; 1.59–2.49), and functional impairment (95% CI, HR 1.40; 1.07–1.83) for BED, and body dissatisfaction (95% CI, HR 1.88; 1.29–2.72) and dieting (95% CI, HR 1.94; 1.35–2.79) for PD. None of the variables most commonly identified as tapping sociocultural pressures related to the thin ideal (eg, thin ideal internalization or positive expectancies about the benefits of thinness) were predictive of ED risk, possibly because they were highly correlated with body dissatisfaction. Consistent with prior studies, body dissatisfaction was a transdiagnostic ED risk factor.

Because many ED risk factors have been shown to be highly collinear,[56] experts have advocated using analytic methods that are suited for handling correlated data and detecting interactions including higher-order interactions among variables, such as classification tree analysis (CTA). Prior studies in ED using CTA included small case samples,[61] cross-sectional data,[62] or symptom-based rather than syndrome-based outcomes.[63] Two studies were identified that used this method for testing for ED. Specifically, in second publication based on the prevention trials data, Stice and colleagues[55] sought to address this gap and found the following. For women with AN (defined in this second publication to include subthreshold cases, resulting in a case sample increased from 9 to 26), a 2-way interaction of low BMI and body dissatisfaction was found, with low BMI at baseline the most potent predictor, followed by body dissatisfaction. CTA identified a complex 4-way interaction for BN. The first partition occurred for high levels of overeating as the most potent predictor, and amplification of this risk from overeating in those women with elevated positive expectancies regarding thinness and body dissatisfaction. Paradoxically, among those with this risk factor combination, lower levels of thin ideal internalization further amplified risk for BN. Regarding, BED, a 4-way interaction was found with elevated body dissatisfaction as the strongest predictor. Risk was amplified by elevated over-eating and low levels of dieting. High levels of thin ideal internalization further amplified risk. For PD, a 3-way interaction was found involving dieting, the strongest predictor, and negative affect and positive thinness internalization, each further amplifying PD risk. Together, these findings suggest both transdiagnostic risk factors and diagnosis-specific risk factors and that ED risk may involve different pathways, or risk subgroups.

Utilizing data on 1297 adolescents (49% male) who participated in a longitudinal cohort study in Australia,[56] risk for ED onset by age 17 or age 20 was examined. Excluding children who had developed an ED before age 14, there were 146 partici-pants (26 boys) with ED onset (no AN). A transdiagnostic ED was created, representing 81 BN, 43 BED, and 22 PD cases. CTA found that the initial split was by gender with ED incident of 18.1% for girls and 4% for boys. For boys, weight/shape concerns at age 14 indicated differential risk as follows: boys with weight/shape concerns in the bottom 12% of normalized scores or between the 12th and 59th percentiles, 1.2% and 1.5%, respectively, developed an ED, compared with 17.1% of boys with elevated weight/shape concerns (top 41% of the sample). For girls, weight/shape con-cerns also were the most potent risk factor and, as for the boys, 3 nonlinear categories were found, each with increasing degrees of risk: among girls in the bottom category, 1.8% developed an ED; among those in a middle category (ranging from the 12th to the 77th percentiles), 8.2% had ED onset; in the upper category, 45.1% of girls devel-oped an ED. Moreover, among girls in the midlevel weight/shape concern group, low externalizing problems were identified to lower risk such that 2.8% had ED onset compared with 12.3% onset among girls with average or above-average externalizing problems. Because the Australian study used a different set of predictor variables (except for BMI and dieting) and focused on a transdiagnosic rather than diagnosis-specific outcome category, these findings cannot be compared directly to the US sample. Weight/shape concern and body dissatisfaction, however, typically are highly correlated. Taken together, consistent with sociocultural explanations, these two studies support the etiologic role of body image concerns in EDs.

Machado and colleagues completed two related case-control studies involving ED patients recruited at specialty treatment centers in Portugal, matching ED cases (*Diagnostic and Statistical Manual of Mental Disorders* [Fourth Edition] [*DSM-IV*]) on demographic variables to healthy controls (HCs) and psychiatric controls (PCs) and examining a large (approximately 120) multifactorial set of risk variables.[53,54] Expo-sure was focused on the time before onset of the first ED symptom of AN or BN, respectively. In both studies, most variables were found not to differentiate ED from HC or PC cases (including several sociocultural factors, such as parental un-employment, parents in risk occupations, and several childhood adversity variables).

Specifically, in a sample of 60 women with BN, compared with 60 HCs,[53] more women with BN reported feeling self-conscious about their physical appearance, negative family experiences related to eating or appearance (undue emphasis on physical appearance, tensions during meals, and comments about weight), appearance-related comments and teasing by friends or others, being overweight as a child or adolescent, feeling fat in childhood, negative feelings about menarche, negative attitudes about parents' weight, childhood anxiety, deliberate self-harm, parental depression, and family difficulties (unresolved disagreements, high parental expectations and criticism, low parental involvement, and feeling inferior to siblings). BN cases also differed significantly from PC (N = 60) on most of these variables. In logistic regressions, two variables were retained for differentiating BN cases versus

HC cases, correctly classifying 93.3% of BN cases and 100% of HC cases: negative attitude about parental weight and childhood overweight. Four variables differentiated BN cases versus PC cases (correct classification: 86.7% BN and 88.3% PC): feeling fat in childhood, deliberate self-harm, unresolved disagreements, and high maternal expectations.

A second case-control study[54] recruited 98 patients with AN, 79 patients with BN, 86 patients with HC, and 68 patients with PC (60 of the BN cases and all HC cases and PC cases were included in the aforementioned study).[53] Compared with HC, women with AN were significantly more likely to report self-consciousness about physical appearance, parental comments about eating, teasing (both unrelated and related to weight/shape), feeling fat in childhood, negative attitudes about parents' weight/shape, a family history of AN or BN, perfectionism, and unresolved family disagreements. Compared with the PC group, women with AN were significantly more likely to report appearance self-consciousness, negative attitudes about parental weight/shape and about menstruation, feeling fat in childhood, a family history of AN or BN, being teased (unrelated to appearance), unresolved family disagreements, and being perfectionistic. Compared with women with AN, women with BN were significantly more likely to report exposure to high parental expectations, family emphasis on fitness, feeling that adolescent overweight conveyed negative consequences, and being overweight in adolescence.

A strength of these studies was the focus on a wide range of potential risk factors. Yet, although the findings from these 2 case-control studies support cultural hypotheses about the role of thinness expectations for girls and women and associated risk factors, such as feeling fat or placing negative valence on overweight in self or others, due to retrospective risk assessment, it cannot be ruled out that patients' current experience of an ED contributed to enhanced or selective recall of body image–related, weight-related, and eating-related experiences. Case matching precluded testing associations between fixed markers and AN or BN. In contrast to research described later, where exposure was measured objectively or using much larger case samples, in these case-control studies, measures of severe adverse childhood events (including bereavement and physical or sexual abuse) were not found associated with AN or BN risk.

Childhood adversity

A Danish register–based study examined exposure (yes/no) before age 6 years to 9 adversity variables in a cohort of all girls born in Denmark to Danish-born parents between 1989 and 2007 (excluding children who died or emigrated before age 6 years) who were followed up to age 25 years. Adversities included family disruption (child not sharing same address with both parents for various reasons), parental somatic illness, residential instability (more than 1 house move between 2 municipalities), parental psychiatric illness, parental substance us disorder, severe parental criminality, parental disability, familial death (loss of a parent or full or half sibling), and placement in foster care. Due to human subjects' concerns, the study did not examine childhood physical abuse or sexual abuse. ED onset was defined as age of first hospitalization for AN, BN, or EDNOS. Of 495,244 girls in the study sample, almost 35% had experienced 1 or more childhood adversities and 2892 (0.58%) were diagnosed with AN and 1027 (0.21%) with BN.

Cumulative incidence of AN was highest for women with no adversity and decreased with increasing number of adversities; AN was associated inversely with severe parental criminality or placement in foster care. In contrast, cumulative incidence of BN was lowest for women with no adversity and increased with increasing number of adversities; family disruption and parental psychiatric illness were significantly associated with BN. In regard to specificity of risk (ED rather than another psychiatric disorder), the study found that exposure to most or all adverse events was associated with increased risk for major mood disorder, anxiety disorder, and obsessive-compulsive disorder. Because hospital-based care is the exception in the treatment of ED and typically connotes greater illness severity,[3,4] it is unclear whether the findings generalize to individuals with no or only outpatient treatment. Nonetheless, the large case samples and objective adversity measures are strengths of this study.

A population-based cohort study using national registries from Denmark and Sweden examined exposure to bereavement from 1 year preconception to 10 years of age as a possible risk factor for broadly defined EDs.[59] Results are described concerning broadly defined AN and BN. Data were extracted for 934,610 girls born in Denmark from 1970 to 2000 and 1,178,146 girls born in Sweden from 1973 to 1997 (excluding girls who had experienced bereavement between ages 10 and 26 years). Girls were followed for 10 years or until they were diagnosed with an ED, emigrated, died, or reached age 26, whichever came first. In all, 64,453 (3.05%) of girls experienced exposure to bereavement, defined as loss of a core relative (prenatal maternal loss of a spouse/child or postnatal loss of a parent or a sibling) or loss of other relatives and by type of death (expected/unexpected). Of the 5878 girls with AN, 166 (2.41%, adjusted incidence rate ratio [IRR] 0.96; 95% CI, 0.82–1.13) were exposed, a nonsignificant association. IRRs also were nonsignificant for timing of exposure, relationship to the deceased, or whether death was expected. Of 1722 girls with BN, 63 were exposed to bereavement. Although the overall association between bereavement and BN status was nonsignificant (adjusted IRR 1.30; 0.97–1.72), the association of bereavement exposure to unexpected death prenatally or postnatally was associated significantly with risk for BN (IRR 2.47; 1.67–3.65).

Using data from a nationally representative sample of US adults (N = 36,309), self-reported exposure before age 18 years to 7 types of childhood maltreatment (harsh physical punishment, physical abuse, sexual abuse, emotional abuse, emotional neglect, physical neglect, and exposure to intimate partner violence) were examined as risk factors for AN, BN, or BED.[57] Among women with AN (N = 240), except for emotional neglect and exposure to partner violence, maltreatment was statistically significant, whereas for men with AN (N = 36), only physical abuse, sexual abuse, and exposure to intimate partner violence were significant predictors. When adjusting for all other forms of maltreatment, in both men and women only the association of sexual abuse and AN diagnosis remained significant. In women with BN (N = 11), sexual abuse, emotional abuse, and emotional neglect were significant; in men (N = 11), associations with BN diagnosis were significant for physical abuse, sexual abuse, emotional neglect, and exposure to intimate partner violence. In fully adjusted models, emotional abuse remained a significant predictor in women with BN; the model could not be calculated for men due to inadequate power and lack of variance. Among women with BED (N = 203), associations were significant for each of the maltreatment categories and, in fully adjusted models, for sexual and emotional abuse. For men (N = 82), sexual abuse and physical neglect were significantly associated with BED; in fully adjusted models, only physical neglect remained significant. Except for exposure to intimate partner violence and physical neglect, which varied by diagnosis and gender, the study suggests that childhood maltreatment is a transdiagnostic and gender-neutral risk factor for AN, BN, and BED.

High-risk environments

Cultural theories have proposed that certain environments confer increased risk for ED development. For example, 1 study provided initial support for a social contagion effect among sororities,[64] but few studies have tested environmental risk hypotheses using systems, rather than individual-level variables. Bould and colleagues[60] addressed this gap with a register-based record linkage study composed of data on 55,059 girls born in Sweden from 1983 and finishing high school in 2002 to 2010, involving 409 schools. Individual-level and school-level variables were measured and individual-level variables were used to estimate odds ratios for different school environment factors and to calculate the contributions of each variable to between-school variation in the incidence of ED at the school level. In all, 2.4% of girls had an ED onset between 16 and 20 years of age; EDs were broadly defined (any *International Classification of Diseases, Tenth Revision* [*ICD-10*] ED code) and extracted from treatment registries. Of the total variation in the odds of ED, 4.4% (95% CI, 2.8–7.1) was due to between-school differences. Individual-level variables with the greatest impact on this variation included parental education, family disposable income, maternal age, having a foreign-born parent, and parental psychiatric history. Models adjusted for individual-level variables and testing the association of school-level variables on variance in the odds of ED found elevated ED risk in schools with a higher proportion of girls or of children of highly educated parents.

SUMMARY

The myriad methodological variations across the 22 studies (including the wide range of risk factors measured) defy reaching straightforward conclusions regarding the role of sociocultural factors in ED risk, with 1 exception. Gender continues to be shown a potent and consistent predictor, although the variations in risk ratios by diagnosis point to the need to focus efforts to improve understanding of risk factors in male populations. Reflecting a major gap, male samples were almost entirely limited to studies reporting on fixed markers and missing from studies that assessed a broad range of variable risk factors. Where included, with notable exceptions of population-based register record linkage studies, boys and men with EDs represented small numbers, underscoring the challenge of studying the etiology of male EDs.

A major novel development in the field is the use and linking of population-based registers, which results in large case samples and provides reliable data on fixed markers or exposure to certain risk factors that may be subject to biased recall. Another novel contribution arises from the application of statistical methods that help address the problem of collinearity of risk variables and elucidate risk subgroups.

Consistent with cultural theories of EDs, body dissatisfaction, or weight concerns, a variable downstream from cultural pressures to achieve a thin beauty ideal was found to increase risk transdiagnostically and across gender groups. In retrospective reports, family or peer pressure about appearance also were significantly associated with risk for AN or BN, although the motivation for such pressure may differ between those 2 diagnostic groups. BMI has been found a bimodal risk factor, with elevated BMI predicting BN or BED and low BMI predicting AN. The literature reviewed further points to the need to continue to focus on diagnosis-specific outcome categories for clarifying ED etiology. Studies of Scandinavian populations identified first-generation immigration status as a protective factor yet also suggest that second-generation immigrants may experience elevated risk for reasons that await further exploration.

Across studies of fixed markers and variable risk factors, findings suggest that beyond the transdiagnostic risk arising from body image concerns, there are disorder-specific risk factors, as exemplified by the role of BMI, immigration status, and childhood aversities. Although most studies included individuals with AN or BN, research of BED and PD continues to lag. Therefore, calls for a transdiagnostic approach to ED classification seem premature.

REFERENCES

1. Adams G, Markus HR. Toward a conception of culture suitable for a social psychology of culture. In: Schaller M, Crandall CS, Schaller M, editors. The psychological foundations of culture. Mahwah (NJ): Lawrence Erlbaum Associates Publishers; 2004. p. 335–60.
2. Striegel-Moore RH, Bulik CM. Risk factors for eating disorders. Am Psychol 2007; 62:181–98.
3. Whiteford H, Weissman RS. Key factors that influence government policies and decision making about healthcare priorities: lessons for the field of eating disorders. Int J Eat Disord 2017;50:315–9.
4. Weissman RS, Rosselli F. Reducing the burden of suffering from eating disorders: unmet treatment needs, cost of illness, and the quest for cost-effectiveness. Behav Res Ther 2017;88:49–64.
5. Pennesi JL, Wade TD. A systematic review of the existing models of disordered eating: do they inform the development of effective interventions? Clin Psychol Rev 2016;43:175–92.
6. Rodin J, Silberstein L, Striegel-Moore R. Women and weight: a normative discontent. Nebr Symp Motiv 1984;32:267–307.
7. Brumberg JJ. Fasting girls: the emergence of anorexia nervosa as a modern disease. Cambridge (MA): Harvard University Press; 1988.
8. Pike KM, Hoek HW, Dunne PE. Cultural trends and eating disorders. Curr Opin Psychiatry 2014;27:436–42.
9. Becker AE. Sociocultural influences on body image and eating disturbance. In: Brownell KD, Walsh BT, Brownell KD, editors. Eating disorders and obesity: a comprehensive handbook. New York: Guilford Press; 2018. p. 127–33.
10. Swami V. Change in risk factors for eating disorder symptomatology in Malay students sojourning in the United Kingdom. Int J Eat Disord 2016;49:695–700.
11. Kolar DR, Rodriguez DL, Chams MM, et al. Epidemiology of eating disorders in Latin America: a systematic review and meta-analysis. Curr Opin Psychiatry 2016;29:363–71.
12. van Hoeken D, Burns JK, Hoek HW. Epidemiology of eating disorders in Africa. Curr Opin Psychiatry 2016;29:372–7.
13. Becker AE, Fay KE, Agnew-Blais J, et al. Social network media exposure and adolescent eating pathology in Fiji. Br J Psychiatry 2011;198:43–50.
14. Hoek HW. Review of the worldwide epidemiology of eating disorders. Curr Opin Psychiatry 2016;29:336–9.
15. Calzo JP, Blashill AJ, Brown TA, et al. Eating disorders and disordered weight and shape control behaviors in sexual minority populations. Curr Psychiatry Rep 2017;19:49.
16. Striegel-Moore RH, Silberstein LR, Rodin J. Toward an understanding of risk factors for bulimia. Am Psychol 1986;41:246–63.
17. Keel PK, Forney KJ. Psychosocial risk factors for eating disorders. Int J Eat Disord 2013;46:433–9.

18. Jacobi C, Hayward C, de Zwaan M, et al. Coming to terms with risk factors for eating disorders: application of risk terminology and suggestions for a general taxonomy. Psychol Bull 2004;130:19–65.
19. Kraemer HC, Kazdin AE, Offord DR, et al. Coming to terms with the terms of risk. Arch Gen Psychiatry 1997;54:337–43.
20. Davis HA, Smith GT. An integrative model of risk for high school disordered eating. J Abnorm Psychol 2018;127:559–70.
21. Schaefer LM, Thompson JK. Self-objectification and disordered eating: a meta-analysis. Int J Eat Disord 2018;51(6):483–502.
22. Velez BL, Campos ID, Moradi B. Relations of sexual objectification and racist discrimination with Latina women's body image and mental health. Couns Psychol 2015;43:906–35.
23. Cheng H-L, Tran AGTT, Miyake ER, et al. Disordered eating among Asian American college women: a racially expanded model of objectification theory. J Couns Psychol 2017;64:179–91.
24. Mustelin L, Hedman AM, Thornton LM, et al. Risk of eating disorders in immigrant populations. Acta Psychiatr Scand 2017;136:156–65.
25. Nakai Y, Nin K, Noma S. Eating disorder symptoms among Japanese female students in 1982, 1992 and 2002. Psychiatry Res 2014;219:151–6.
26. Stice E, Gau JM, Rohde P, et al. Risk factors that predict future onset of each DSM-5 eating disorder: Predictive specificity in high-risk adolescent females. J Abnorm Psychol 2017;126:38–51.
27. Bakalar JL, Shank LM, Vannucci A, et al. Recent advances in developmental and risk factor research on eating disorders. Curr Psychiatry Rep 2015;17:42.
28. Culbert KM, Racine SE, Klump KL. Research review: what we have learned about the causes of eating disorders - a synthesis of sociocultural, psychological, and biological research. J Child Psychol Psychiatry 2015;56:1141–64.
29. Schaumberg K, Jangmo A, Thornton LM, et al. Patterns of diagnostic transition in eating disorders: a longitudinal population study in Sweden. Psychol Med 2018;1–9 [Epub ahead of print].
30. Welch E, Jangmo A, Thornton LM, et al. Treatment-seeking patients with binge-eating disorder in the Swedish national registers: clinical course and psychiatric comorbidity. BMC Psychiatry 2016;16:163.
31. Udo T, Grilo CM. Prevalence and correlates of DSM-5-defined eating disorders in a nationally representative sample of U.S. adults. Biol Psychiatry 2018;84:345–54.
32. Nagl M, Jacobi C, Paul M, et al. Prevalence, incidence, and natural course of anorexia and bulimia nervosa among adolescents and young adults. Eur Child Adolesc Psychiatry 2016;25:903–18.
33. Mustelin L, Bulik CM, Kaprio J, et al. Prevalence and correlates of binge eating disorder related features in the community. Appetite 2017;109:165–71.
34. Striegel-Moore RH, Franko DL. Should binge eating disorder be included in the DSM-V? A critical review of the state of the evidence. Annu Rev Clin Psychol 2008;4:305–24.
35. Schluter N, Schmidt R, Kittel R, et al. Loss of control eating in adolescents from the community. Int J Eat Disord 2016;49:413–20.
36. Watson HJ, Joyce T, French E, et al. Prevention of eating disorders: A systematic review of randomized, controlled trials. Int J Eat Disord 2016;49:833–62.
37. Le LK, Barendregt JJ, Hay P, et al. Prevention of eating disorders: a systematic review and meta-analysis. Clin Psychol Rev 2017;53:46–58.

38. Smink FRE, van Hoeken D, Dijkstra JK, et al. Self-esteem and peer-perceived social status in early adolescence and prediction of eating pathology in young adulthood. Int J Eat Disord 2018;51(8):852–62.
39. Micali N, Martini MG, Thomas JJ, et al. Lifetime and 12-month prevalence of eating disorders amongst women in mid-life: a population-based study of diagnoses and risk factors. BMC Med 2017;15:12.
40. Mustelin L, Silen Y, Raevuori A, et al. The DSM-5 diagnostic criteria for anorexia nervosa may change its population prevalence and prognostic value. J Psychiatr Res 2016;77:85–91.
41. Mohler-Kuo M, Schnyder U, Dermota P, et al. The prevalence, correlates, and help-seeking of eating disorders in Switzerland. Psychol Med 2016;46:2749–58.
42. Solmi F, Hotopf M, Hatch SL, et al. Eating disorders in a multi-ethnic inner-city UK sample: prevalence, comorbidity and service use. Soc Psychiatry Psychiatr Epidemiol 2016;51:369–81.
43. Hammerle F, Huss M, Ernst V, et al. Thinking dimensional: prevalence of DSM-5 early adolescent full syndrome, partial and subthreshold eating disorders in a cross-sectional survey in German schools. BMJ Open 2016;6:e010843.
44. Benjet C, Borges G, Mendez E, et al. Eight-year incidence of psychiatric disorders and service use from adolescence to early adulthood: longitudinal follow-up of the Mexican Adolescent Mental Health Survey. Eur Child Adolesc Psychiatry 2016;25:163–73.
45. O'Brien KM, Whelan DR, Sandler DP, et al. Predictors and long-term health outcomes of eating disorders. PLoS One 2017;12:e0181104.
46. Razaz N, Cnattingius S. Association between maternal body mass index in early pregnancy and anorexia nervosa in daughters. Int J Eat Disord 2018;51(8):906–13.
47. Sundquist J, Ohlsson H, Sundquist K, et al. Common adult psychiatric disorders in Swedish primary care where most mental health patients are treated. BMC Psychiatry 2017;17:235.
48. Hvelplund C, Hansen BM, Koch SV, et al. Perinatal risk factors for feeding and eating disorders in children aged 0 to 3 years. Pediatrics 2016;137:e20152575.
49. Lewer M, Bauer A, Hartmann AS, et al. Different facets of body image disturbance in binge eating disorder: a review. Nutrients 2017;9 [pii:E1294].
50. Volpe U, Tortorella A, Manchia M, et al. Eating disorders: what age at onset? Psychiatry Res 2016;238:225–7.
51. Becker CB, Middlemass K, Taylor B, et al. Food insecurity and eating disorder pathology. Int J Eat Disord 2017;50:1031–40.
52. Bryant-Waugh R, Markham L, Kreipe RE, et al. Feeding and eating disorders in childhood. Int J Eat Disord 2010;43:98–111.
53. Goncalves S, Machado BC, Martins C, et al. Retrospective correlates for bulimia nervosa: a matched case-control study. Eur Eat Disord Rev 2016;24:197–205.
54. Machado BC, Goncalves SF, Martins C, et al. Anorexia nervosa versus bulimia nervosa: differences based on retrospective correlates in a case-control study. Eat Weight Disord 2016;21:185–97.
55. Stice E, Desjardins CD. Interactions between risk factors in the prediction of onset of eating disorders: exploratory hypothesis generating analyses. Behav Res Ther 2018;105:52–62.
56. Allen KL, Byrne SM, Crosby RD, et al. Testing for interactive and non-linear effects of risk factors for binge eating and purging eating disorders. Behav Res Ther 2016;87:40–7.

57. Afifi TO, Sareen J, Fortier J, et al. Child maltreatment and eating disorders among men and women in adulthood: results from a nationally representative united states sample. Int J Eat Disord 2018;50(11):1281–96.
58. Larsen JT, Munk-Olsen T, Bulik CM, et al. Early childhood adversities and risk of eating disorders in women: a Danish register-based cohort study. Int J Eat Disord 2017;50:1404–12.
59. Su X, Liang H, Yuan W, et al. Prenatal and early life stress and risk of eating disorders in adolescent girls and young women. Eur Child Adolesc Psychiatry 2016; 25:1245–53.
60. Bould H, De Stavola B, Magnusson C, et al. The influence of school on whether girls develop eating disorders. Int J Epidemiol 2016;45:480–8.
61. Striegel-Moore RH, Dohm FA, Kraemer HC, et al. Risk factors for binge-eating disorders: an exploratory study. Int J Eat Disord 2007;40:481–7.
62. Racine SE, VanHuysse JL, Keel PK, et al. Eating disorder-specific risk factors moderate the relationship between negative urgency and binge eating: a behavioral genetic investigation. J Abnorm Psychol 2017;126:481–94.
63. Fairweather-Schmidt AK, Wade TD. Weight-related peer-teasing moderates genetic and environmental risk and disordered eating: twin study. Br J Psychiatry 2017;210:350–5.
64. Crandall CS. Social contagion of binge eating. J Pers Soc Psychol 1988;55: 588–98.

Other Topics

Body Image in the Context of Eating Disorders

Siân A. McLean, PhD[a],*, Susan J. Paxton, PhD[b]

KEYWORDS

- Body dissatisfaction • Eating disorders • Overvaluation of weight and shape
- Prevention • Treatment

KEY POINTS

- Body dissatisfaction may be present in all genders and across the lifespan, and is associated with considerable distress and quality of life impairment.
- Body image constructs including overvaluation of weight and shape, fear of weight gain, and preoccupation with weight and shape constitute core eating disorder psychopathology.
- Addressing body dissatisfaction is an essential element of eating disorders treatment and is important for reducing risk of relapse.
- Future directions for intervention require expanded reach to meet the needs of underserved populations, such as men, and people with higher body weight.

INTRODUCTION

Body image has been described as a multidimensional construct that encompasses the internalized view one has of one's body.[1] It includes perceptions, thoughts, feelings, and attitudes related to physical aspects of the body, such as weight and shape, leanness and muscularity, athleticism, sexual attractiveness, physical function, and aging.[2] Although the concept of body image is broad, there has been a focus in research and practice on appearance-related self-perceptions, thoughts, feelings, and attitudes because these have been linked most frequently to negative psychological outcomes. For similar reasons, although body image lies on a continuum from positive feelings of appreciation and enjoyment to negative feelings of loathing and distress, until recently, the focus of research and practice has primarily been on negative body image experiences. This article uses the widely accepted term of "body dissatisfaction" to describe negative conceptualizations of body image, especially

Disclosure Statement: Neither of the authors has any disclosures.
[a] Institute for Health and Sport, Victoria University, Ballarat Road, Footscray, Melbourne, Victoria 8001, Australia; [b] Department of Psychology and Counselling, School of Psychology and Public Health, La Trobe University, Melbourne, Victoria 3086, Australia
* Corresponding author.
E-mail address: sian.mclean@vu.edu.au

Psychiatr Clin N Am 42 (2019) 145–156
https://doi.org/10.1016/j.psc.2018.10.006
0193-953X/19/© 2018 Elsevier Inc. All rights reserved.

psych.theclinics.com

related to appearance. The article reviews the prevalence and consequences of body dissatisfaction and models of body dissatisfaction development. The experience of different facets of body image within eating disorders, and prevention, and early intervention and treatment approaches for body dissatisfaction are outlined. The discussion of body dissatisfaction excludes reference to body dysmorphic disorder, which is beyond the scope of this article.

Body dissatisfaction may be present in men and women, and boys and girls, although the source of body dissatisfaction typically differs. In women and girls, body dissatisfaction usually relates to concerns about weight and shape, particularly a desire to be thinner, whereas in men and boys, it generally relates to concerns about being insufficiently lean or muscular.[2] Although potentially present in both genders and at all life stages including childhood and midlife, body dissatisfaction most frequently develops during adolescence[3] and is more prevalent in women and girls. In a large survey of adults, moderate to marked body dissatisfaction was reported by 33.0% of women and 15.2% of men.[4]

THE NEGATIVE IMPACT OF BODY DISSATISFACTION

The negative consequences of high levels of body dissatisfaction are increasingly evident. Body dissatisfaction is associated with distress and impaired physical and psychosocial quality of life.[4] Although body dissatisfaction occurs more frequently in women than men, the strength of adverse association between quality of life impairment and body dissatisfaction is more pronounced in men.[4] In addition, body dissatisfaction predicts the development of low self-esteem and depressive symptoms in adolescents[5] and a range of unhealthy behaviors including onset of regular smoking[6] and unsafe sexual behaviors.[7]

Not surprisingly, body dissatisfaction predicts attempts to change the body through use of extreme weight loss or muscle building behaviors.[8] Body dissatisfaction and unhealthy dieting have also been observed to predict the development of overweight and obesity in girls, although the mechanisms involved are not entirely clear.[9] More readily understood is the consistently observed predictive relationship between body dissatisfaction and disordered eating and clinical eating disorders. Body dissatisfaction, with a focus on weight and shape concerns, has been identified as among the most potent and best replicated risk factors for bulimia nervosa (BN) and to a lesser extent anorexia nervosa (AN).[10] In light of the high frequency and profoundly negative impact of body dissatisfaction, a deeper understanding of its causes and the need for effective interventions is warranted.

MODELS OF DEVELOPMENT OF BODY DISSATISFACTION

Several models have been proposed to explain the development of body dissatisfaction but three have been most prominent: (1) the sociocultural model or tripartite influence model[1]; (2) extension of this model, the biopsychosocial model[11]; and (3) objectification theory.[12,13] There is empirical support for each of these models.

The sociocultural model emphasizes the influence on body image of three sociocultural sources of appearance pressure: (1) media, (2) family, and (3) peers.[1] When an individual experiences pressure to conform to unrealistic appearance ideals from one or more of these sources, it is proposed that these ideals are internalized and the appearance ideal becomes a personal goal or value to which to aspire (described as internalization of the appearance ideal). This contributes to an elevated focus on appearance and, in particular, to an increase in upward body comparison (comparison of one's appearance with perceived positive appearance qualities of others). Because individuals seldom perceive themselves as living up to their ideals or to meet the standards of comparison targets, body dissatisfaction follows. This model has received cross-sectional and prospective empirical support from numerous studies of adolescents and young adults.[14,15]

The biopsychosocial model of the development of body dissatisfaction extends on the sociocultural model by including biological and psychological variables as risk factors for body dissatisfaction.[11] Biological risk factors include proposed genetic influences[16] and larger body size,[17] which in a social environment highly critical of larger body size is proposed to result in self-criticism and body dissatisfaction. Psychological factors postulated to increase risk of body dissatisfaction include negative affect, low self-esteem, and perfectionism. In this model, negative affect increases negative attributional bias and thus the likelihood of evaluating one's own body negatively.[18] Low self-esteem may similarly contribute to a negative view of one's body, but it has also been proposed to increase vulnerability to internalization of appearance ideals and upward appearance comparisons.[11] In relation to perfectionism, it has been suggested that individuals who are perfectionistic and apply inflexible evaluative criteria to themselves may apply these same criteria to achieving the perfect body, which being rarely achievable contributes to body dissatisfaction.[19] There is strong evidence to support the inclusion of low self-esteem and depressive symptoms in predictive models of body dissatisfaction,[5,11,18] although this is not consistently the case.[20] Empirical research into the role of perfectionism is still in early stages.[19,21]

Objectification theory[12] is based on the premise that in Western societies, the female body (and increasingly the male body), is viewed as an object to be looked at and evaluated according to appearance.[13] Through this experience, individuals learn to internalize an observer's perspective on their own body and to evaluate it relative to prevailing social ideals. It is proposed that this self-objectification leads to body shame because of perceived failure to live up to the social appearance ideal, and increased body surveillance, and consequently body dissatisfaction.[13] In samples of women and men, there is considerable correlational support for relationships within this model (eg, see Ref.[22]). Although prospective research is still in early stages, self-objectification has been found to predict later appearance concerns in adolescent boys and girls.[23] Some experimental research indicates that when self-objectification is increased, negative attitudes toward one's body also increase in women and men.[24,25] Attention is now being focused on self-objectification in online and social media contexts. Online self-presentation of one's image provides a platform through which individuals may be objectified by others, further reinforcing self-objectification. Research has shown that online self-presentation increases self-objectification in young women[26]; however, the extent to which this process influences body dissatisfaction is yet to be investigated.

Collectively, these models indicate a range of sociocultural and psychological factors that are implicated in the development of body dissatisfaction. Understanding how these factors individually and cumulatively increase risk for and maintain experiences of body dissatisfaction provides guidance for identifying targets for prevention and treatment. These are described further next in relation to approaches to intervention for body dissatisfaction within eating disorder treatment.

THE EXPERIENCE OF BODY IMAGE IN EATING DISORDERS

In addition to being a risk factor for the development of eating disorders, body dissatisfaction and related experiences constitute key diagnostic criteria for AN and BN. However, not all eating disorders include body dissatisfaction or related disturbances as diagnostic criteria. Avoidant/restrictive food intake disorder, feeding and eating disorder not elsewhere classified, and binge eating disorder do not feature body image–related diagnostic criteria.[27] Despite the absence of body image–related criteria for binge eating disorder, scholars argue that overvaluation of weight and shape not only provides important information about binge eating disorder severity, but also has diagnostic relevance.[28] Indeed, overvaluation of weight and shape and their control is considered to be a core psychopathological feature across eating disorders within the transdiagnostic formulation of eating disorders.[29]

Conceptualizations of overvaluation of shape and weight within theoretical models and treatment formulations typically focus on overvaluation of the thin-body ideal and have emerged from research and clinical observations with girls and women. However, the general concept of overvaluation of appearance likely also has relevance for men and boys. Body concerns for men and boys have been described as having a dual focus on the muscular and lean appearance ideal.[30] It is proposed that overvaluation of this dual-focused appearance ideal drives distinct disordered behaviors, such as overconsumption of protein and excessive weight training, and extreme restriction of calories and dietary fat intake, in pursuit of a muscular and lean physique, respectively.[30] Support for this proposition has been found in cross-sectional modeling of men's body concerns whereby direct pathways from muscularity dissatisfaction to engagement in muscularity-enhancing behavior and from body fat dissatisfaction to weight-controlling disordered eating behaviors were observed.[31]

Although disturbances in body image are represented in the diagnostic criteria of AN and BN, the contribution of specific aspects of body image disturbance differ according to diagnosis. This is consistent with recent research in which body image constructs, such as body dissatisfaction, fear of weight gain, preoccupation with weight and shape, and overvaluation of weight and shape, are recognized as being distinct from one another and also as having distinct relationships with core eating disorder symptoms in nonclinical samples of adolescents and clinical samples of patients with eating disorders.[32–34] Where direct comparisons across studies could be made, dietary restraint was related to preoccupation with weight and shape in adolescent girls and boys and patients with binge eating disorder, but not patients with AN, and to overvaluation of weight and shape in adolescent boys but not patients with either AN or binge eating disorder. Furthermore, binge eating was related to overvaluation in boys and to body dissatisfaction and preoccupation in girls in the adolescent sample, but was not related to any body image constructs in patients with binge eating disorder.[32–34] The greatest similarities across samples appeared for relationships with broader psychological outcomes, distress, or depression symptoms, whereby in all samples, overvaluation and preoccupation were uniquely related to higher symptomatology. Comparisons among samples are somewhat limited by lack of consistency in inclusion of body image constructs and eating disorder symptoms.

Network analyses also facilitate understanding of the interrelationships between body image constructs and eating disorder symptoms. The representation of symptoms, such as body dissatisfaction, fear of weight gain, and preoccupation with shape and weight, as unique constructs with distinct relationships to eating behaviors is supported by this emerging research. For example, in a network analysis of symptoms of BN within a clinical sample, body dissatisfaction was directly related to vomiting, a compensatory behavior in BN, and fear of weight gain was revealed to be a core symptom of BN.[35] Similarly, in a nonclinical sample of college-age women, fear of weight gain was found to be associated with thoughts of purging, and guilt after overeating.[36] Furthermore, in a transdiagnostic sample, overvaluation of weight and shape was found to be central to the symptom network, regardless of eating disorder diagnosis.[37] The presence of and consistency of these interrelationships in clinical and nonclinical samples suggests the utility of these body image constructs as targets for prevention and early intervention in eating disorders.

BODY IMAGE IN THE RECOVERY FROM EATING DISORDERS

It is increasingly being recognized that effectively treating body image disturbances is likely to be an essential aspect of treatment of eating disorders. Pennesi and Wade[38] recently reviewed existing theoretic models of disordered eating and concluded that negative body image constructs (eg, weight and shape concerns and body dissatisfaction) emerged as a common risk factor across the major theoretic models examined and suggested addressing body image may be a pivotal therapeutic component of future effective interventions. In addition, empirical analyses have identified body dissatisfaction as an important maintaining factor once an eating disorder has been established[39] and an important factor predicting risk of relapse following eating disorders treatment.[40]

Recent analyses of body image and treatment outcome data from the Anorexia Nervosa Treatment Outpatient Study (ANTOP) provide empirical support for the proposal that body image concerns play a key role in maintaining this disorder.[41] In this large, multicenter study comparing outcomes from three different outpatient psychotherapeutic treatments, greater body image disturbance at treatment commencement predicted perceived stress during psychotherapy, which in turn predicted depressive symptoms at the end of therapy, which in turn predicted poorer body mass index and disordered eating symptoms at 1-year follow-up.[41] The authors concluded that these findings suggest that body image interventions during treatment of AN are likely to be beneficial, but they do warn against interventions that may increase the stress experienced by patients in light of the pathway from greater stress to more negative treatment outcomes.[41]

Further support for a key role for body image concerns in the maintenance of AN is provided by research conducted by Calugi and colleagues.[42] The authors examined outcomes at 12-month follow-up in patients with AN who received inpatient enhanced cognitive behavioral therapy[29] and found that baseline and end-of-therapy scores on measures of body image concerns predicted positive body mass index outcomes. The authors conclude, "This confirms the need to monitor body image concern, and suggests that strategies and procedures designed to improve this feature during treatment should be enhanced in patients with anorexia nervosa."[42(p67)]

INTERVENTION AND TREATMENT FOR BODY DISSATISFACTION

Intervention for body dissatisfaction can take the form of prevention, early intervention, and treatment of clinically severe body dissatisfaction independent of eating disorders, or as described previously in relation to recovery from eating disorders. The selection of a particular type of intervention depends on the specific constellation and severity of symptoms. **Fig. 1** shows intervention strategies to address risk and maintenance factors for body dissatisfaction and thereby build body acceptance.

Prevention of Body Dissatisfaction

Prevention programs are frequently delivered to groups rather than individually, and either target populations who are asymptomatic, but because of demographic characteristics, such as age and gender, are at higher risk of developing body dissatisfaction (universal or selective prevention interventions) or target individuals within at-risk populations who have elevated levels of body dissatisfaction but have not yet reached

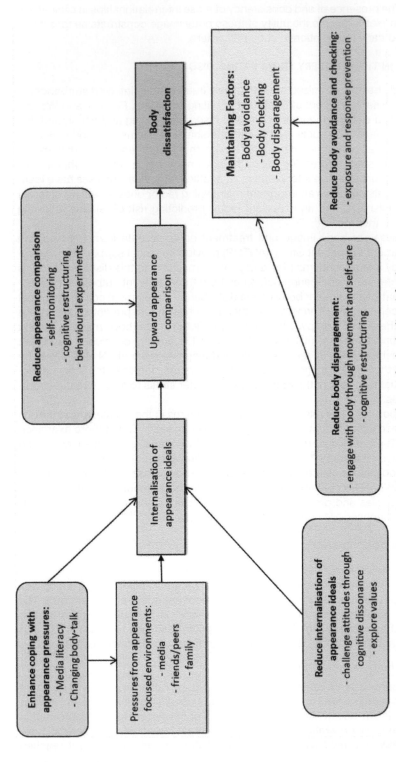

Fig. 1. Schematic of interventions addressing risk and maintaining factors for body dissatisfaction.

threshold criteria for an eating disorder (indicated prevention interventions). Delivery settings are typically schools (eg, see Refs.[43-45]) and universities.[46] These settings are appropriate for group delivery of prevention because intact groups for program delivery may already be established, they present opportunities for developmentally appropriate intervention material, and are also environments in which sustained inter- action and learning opportunities can be integrated in the broader context of the setting.[47]

Prevention approaches target modifiable risk factors for body dissatisfaction with a focus on appearance pressures from social sources including family, peers, and me- dia; internalization of appearance ideals; and upward appearance comparisons, as shown in **Fig. 1** (eg, see Refs.[48,49]). Some programs aim to assist participants to change their immediate appearance environment by learning through role-plays to change the negative direction of peer appearance conversations and to reduce appearance teasing.[45,48] A well-supported strategy is to help build coping strategies in relation to environmental pressures and, in particular, to build skills to critically analyze and evaluate appearance media (ie, enhancing media literacy).[44,45] Recent research has extended prevention interventions to address the negative impact of so- cial media with the use of social media literacy (building skills to analyze and evaluate social media especially content on social networking sites).[50]

Other strategies have specifically addressed internalization of appearance ideals. Cognitive dissonance is the strategy that has most research support and is one in which participants, usually individuals with existing body image concerns, engage in activities in which they challenge the appearance ideal and thereby challenge their own values.[46] Finally, prevention approaches include the examination of core values and exploring where meeting appearance ideals fits within one's values. This strategy generally helps to reduce the prioritization given to meeting appearance ideals.[49,50]

Early Intervention and Treatment

Early intervention and treatment of body dissatisfaction are distinguishable mainly by the stage of illness or level of symptom development at which intervention is provided rather than the specific therapeutic techniques used. Consequently, these are described together. In addition, interventions for stand-alone body image problems are similar to those incorporated into eating disorder treatment. Despite body image disturbances being recognized as central to the experience of and treatment of eating disorders, in relation to delivering cognitive behavior therapy for eating disorders, cli- nicians have reported being most worried about working with body image issues.[51] Thus, additional guidance and supervision for body dissatisfaction interventions may be required.

Similar to prevention, early intervention and treatment address factors shown to contribute to the development of body dissatisfaction. However, in addition to factors that convey risk, factors that maintain the experience of body dissatisfaction are also included in treatment approaches.[29,52-54] These include body avoidance and check- ing behaviors and ongoing body disparagement.[55] Furthermore, treatment is typically couched within a therapeutic model, the most frequently evaluated treatment model for body dissatisfaction being cognitive behavioral therapy.[56]

Body avoidance behaviors include avoiding mirrors, or avoiding situations in which a person believes their appearance will be observed and scrutinized, and wearing oversized clothing to camouflage the body.[57] It is proposed that these behaviors main- tain body dissatisfaction by preventing the individual from disconfirming irrational be- liefs about their weight and shape.[58] Body checking behaviors are repeated behaviors aimed at assessing one's shape or weight, such as weighing or other measurement strategies, and are proposed to maintain body dissatisfaction and eating disordered behaviors by increasing attention to disliked parts of the body thereby increasing body dissatisfaction.[57] Patients frequently move between avoidance and checking.

To address body avoidance behaviors, graded exposure approaches are frequently used. In particular, graded mirror and video exposure have been found to be effective in reducing body dissatisfaction, particularly in patients with an eating disorder (eg, see Ref.[59]). Body checking has been effectively addressed using behavioral techniques including stimulus control and exposure response prevention and these have been shown to reduce body dissatisfaction in clinical and nonclinical samples.[56]

Interventions often aim to provide skills to identify the presence and frequency of the negative cognitive behavior of upward appearance comparison through self-monitoring. Cognitive restructuring and behavioral experiment techniques are then implemented to reduce the frequency of engagement in and negative emotional consequences that result from upward appearance comparison.[55]

Finally, approaches to address body disparagement are important for body dissatisfaction treatment. Body disparagement refers to the tendency for individuals with body dissatisfaction to denigrate their bodies or to disengage from body interactions, and for some, disparagement is experienced as intense body loathing.[29]

Reengaging with positive body experiences, particularly nonappearance or functional aspects body experience, through self-care and movement, and cognitive restructuring of denigrating self-talk aim to open a new relationship and way of relating to the body that is less focused on appearance and less self-critical.[55] Yoga interventions and self-compassion therapy are examples of these approaches and initial findings suggest these have promise for body dissatisfaction intervention.[60,61]

FUTURE DIRECTIONS

Despite recent improvements in outcomes from evaluation of prevention programs, particularly for individuals already exhibiting some signs of body dissatisfaction,[47] gaps in application and evaluation have been identified. Specifically, application to a wider age range and wider spectrum of body concerns,[62] and greater length of follow-up, have been recommended.[47] Partially responding to these gaps, and also recognizing newly emerging pressures on appearance and treatment approaches, future directions for prevention programs have incorporated novel intervention approaches, such as mindfulness and self-compassion,[63] social media literacy,[50] use of technology through mobile-apps,[64] task-shifting delivery to nonexpert facilitators,[43] and adaptation of cognitive dissonance programs for men.[65] These approaches have shown promise, but further research is necessary to establish more robust evidence of their impact.

Similarly, body image–specific interventions demonstrate positive outcomes in stand-alone or eating disorders treatment contexts as reviewed previously. However, it is also apparent that there is a need to build further evidence of effectiveness in other populations, including men, and people of higher body weights. This is important in light of the greater recognition of the growing prevalence of muscularity-oriented body dissatisfaction and disordered eating in men,[30] and identification of overvaluation of shape and weight as a core psychopathological feature of binge eating disorder,[28] and recognition of diagnoses in people at higher body weights, and with a history of higher body weight.[66] Expanding prevention and treatment through novel approaches, and to meet the needs of underrepresented populations will significantly enhance the benefit to individuals with body dissatisfaction.

REFERENCES

1. Thompson JK, Heinberg LJ, Altabe M, et al. Exacting beauty: theory, assessment, and treatment of body image disturbance. Washington, DC: American Psychological Association; 1999.
2. Grogan S. Body image: understanding body dissatisfaction in men, women and children. 3rd edition. Abingdon (United Kingdom): Routledge; 2017.
3. Rohde P, Stice E, Marti CN. Development and predictive effects of eating disorder risk factors during adolescence: implications for prevention efforts. Int J Eat Disord 2015;48:187–98.
4. Griffiths S, Hay P, Mitchison D, et al. Sex differences in the relationships between body dissatisfaction, quality of life and psychological distress. Aust N Z J Public Health 2016;40:518–22.
5. Paxton SJ, Eisenberg ME, Neumark-Sztainer D. Prospective predictors of body dissatisfaction in adolescent girls and boys: a five-year longitudinal study. Dev Psychol 2006;42:888–99.
6. Kaufman AR, Augustson EM. Predictors of regular cigarette smoking among adolescent females: does body image matter? Nicotine Tob Res 2008;10:1301–9.
7. Schooler D. Early adolescent body image predicts subsequent condom use behavior among girls. Sex Res Social Policy 2013;10:52–61.
8. Neumark-Sztainer D, Paxton SJ, Hannan PJ, et al. Does body satisfaction matter? Five-year longitudinal associations between body satisfaction and health behaviors in adolescent females and males. J Adolesc Health 2006;39:244–51.
9. Haines J, Kleinman KP, Rifas-Shiman SL, et al. Examination of shared risk and protective factors for overweight and disordered eating among adolescents. Arch Pediatr Adolesc Med 2010;164:336–43.
10. Stice E, Gau JM, Rohde P, et al. Risk factors that predict future onset of each DSM–5 eating disorder: predictive specificity in high-risk adolescent females. J Abnorm Psychol 2017;126:38–51.
11. Rodgers RF, Paxton SJ, McLean SA. A biopsychosocial model of body image concerns and disordered eating in early adolescent girls. J Youth Adolesc 2014;43:814–23.
12. Fredrickson BL, Roberts T-A. Objectification theory: toward understanding women's lived experiences and mental health risks. Psychol Women Q 1997; 21:173–206.
13. Tiggemann M. Objectification theory: of relevance for eating disorder researchers and clinicians? Clin Psychol 2013;17:35–45.
14. Rodgers RF, McLean SA, Paxton SJ. Longitudinal relationships among internalization of the media ideal, peer social comparison, and body dissatisfaction: implications for the tripartite influence model. Dev Psychol 2015;51:706–13.
15. Yamamiya Y, Shroff H, Thompson JK. The tripartite influence model of body image and eating disturbance: a replication with a Japanese sample. Int J Eat Disord 2008;41:88–91.
16. Suisman J, Klump K. Genetic and neuroscientific perspectives on body image. In: Cash TF, Smolak L, editors. Body image: a handbook of science, practice, and prevention. 2nd edition. New York: Guilford press; 2011. p. 29–38.
17. Paxton SJ, Neumark-Sztainer D, Hannan PJ, et al. Body dissatisfaction prospectively predicts depressive mood and low self-esteem in adolescent girls and boys. J Clin Child Adolesc Psychol 2006;35:539–49.
18. Bearman SK, Presnell K, Martinez E, et al. The skinny on body dissatisfaction: a longitudinal study of adolescent girls and boys. J Youth Adolesc 2006;35:229–41.

19. Boone L, Soenens B, Luyten P. When or why does perfectionism translate into eating disorder pathology? A longitudinal examination of the moderating and mediating role of body dissatisfaction. J Abnorm Psychol 2014;123:412–8.
20. Wojtowicz AE, von Ranson KM. Weighing in on risk factors for body dissatisfaction: a one-year prospective study of middle-adolescent girls. Body Image 2012;9:20–30.
21. Nichols TE, Damiano SR, Gregg K, et al. Psychological predictors of body image attitudes and concerns in young children. Body Image 2018;27:10–20.
22. Manago AM, Ward L, Lemm KM, et al. Facebook involvement, objectified body consciousness, body shame, and sexual assertiveness in college women and men. Sex Roles 2015;72:1–14.
23. Dakanalis A, Carrà G, Calogero R, et al. The developmental effects of media-ideal internalization and self-objectification processes on adolescents' negative body-feelings, dietary restraint, and binge eating. Eur Child Adolesc Psychiatry 2015;24:997–1010.
24. Aubrey JS, Henson J, Hopper KM, et al. A picture is worth twenty words (about the self): testing the priming influence of visual sexual objectification on women's self-objectification. Commun Res Rep 2009;26:271–84.
25. Hebl MR, King EB, Lin J. The swimsuit becomes us all: ethnicity, gender, and vulnerability to self-objectification. Pers Soc Psychol Bull 2004;30:1322–31.
26. de Vries DA, Peter J. Women on display: the effect of portraying the self online on women's self-objectification. Comput Hum Behav 2013;29:1483–9.
27. Thomas JJ, Hartmann AS, Killgore WDS. Non-fat-phobic eating disorders: why we need to investigate implicit associations and neural correlates. Int J Eat Disord 2013;46:416–9.
28. Grilo CM, Masheb RM, White MA. Significance of overvaluation of shape/weight in binge-eating disorder: comparative study with overweight and bulimia nervosa. Obesity (Silver Spring) 2010;18:499–504.
29. Fairburn CG. Cognitive behavior therapy and eating disorders. New York: Guilford; 2008.
30. Lavender JM, Brown TA, Murray SB. Men, muscles, and eating disorders: an overview of traditional and muscularity-oriented disordered eating. Curr Psychiatry Rep 2017;19:32.
31. Tylka TL. Refinement of the tripartite influence model for men: dual body image pathways to body change behaviors. Body Image 2011;8:199–207.
32. Linardon J, Phillipou A, Castle D, et al. The relative associations of shape and weight over-evaluation, preoccupation, dissatisfaction, and fear of weight gain with measures of psychopathology: AN extension study in individuals with anorexia nervosa. Eat Behav 2018;29:54–8.
33. Lydecker JA, White MA, Grilo CM. Form and formulation: examining the distinctiveness of body image constructs in treatment-seeking patients with binge-eating disorder. J Consult Clin Psychol 2017;85:1095–103.
34. Mitchison D, Hay P, Griffiths S, et al. Disentangling body image: the relative associations of overvaluation, dissatisfaction, and preoccupation with psychological distress and eating disorder behaviors in male and female adolescents. Int J Eat Disord 2017;50:118–26.
35. Levinson CA, Zerwas S, Calebs B, et al. The core symptoms of bulimia nervosa, anxiety, and depression: a network analysis. J Abnorm Psychol 2017;126:340–54.
36. Rodgers RF, DuBois R, Frumkin MR, et al. A network approach to eating disorder symptomatology: do desire for thinness and fear of gaining weight play unique roles in the network? Body Image 2018;27:1–9.

37. DuBois RH, Rodgers RF, Franko DL, et al. A network analysis investigation of the cognitive-behavioral theory of eating disorders. Behav Res Ther 2017;97:213–21.
38. Pennesi J-L, Wade TD. A systematic review of the existing models of disordered eating: do they inform the development of effective interventions? Clin Psychol Rev 2016;43:175–92.
39. Stice E, Shaw HE. Role of body dissatisfaction in the onset and maintenance of eating pathology: a synthesis of research findings. J Psychosom Res 2002;53: 985–93.
40. Dingemans AE, van Son GE, Aardoom JJ, et al. Predictors of psychological outcome in patients with eating disorders: a routine outcome monitoring study. Int J Eat Disord 2016;49:863–73.
41. Junne F, Wild B, Resmark G, et al. The importance of body image disturbances for the outcome of outpatient psychotherapy in patients with anorexia nervosa: results of the ANTOP-study. Eur Eat Disord Rev 2018. https://doi.org/10.1002/erv.2623.
42. Calugi S, El Ghoch M, Conti M, et al. Preoccupation with shape or weight, fear of weight gain, feeling fat and treatment outcomes in patients with anorexia nervosa: a longitudinal study. Behav Res Ther 2018;105:63–8.
43. Diedrichs PC, Atkinson MJ, Steer RJ, et al. Effectiveness of a brief school-based body image intervention 'Dove Confident Me: single Session' when delivered by teachers and researchers: results from a cluster randomised controlled trial. Behav Res Ther 2015;74:94–104.
44. McLean SA, Wertheim EH, Marques MD, et al. Dismantling prevention: comparison of outcomes following media literacy and appearance comparison modules in a randomised controlled trial. J Health Psychol 2016. https://doi.org/10.1177/1359105316678668. Advance online publication.
45. Wilksch SM, Paxton SJ, Byrne SM, et al. Prevention Across the Spectrum: a randomized controlled trial of three programs to reduce risk factors for both eating disorders and obesity. Psychol Med 2015;45:1811–23.
46. Stice E, Rohde P, Durant S, et al. Effectiveness of peer-led dissonance-based eating disorder prevention groups: results from two randomized pilot trials. Behav Res Ther 2013;51:197–206.
47. Yager Z, Diedrichs PC, Ricciardelli LA, et al. What works in secondary schools? A systematic review of classroom-based body image programs. Body Image 2013; 10:271–81.
48. Dunstan CJ, Paxton SJ, McLean SA. An evaluation of a body image intervention in adolescent girls delivered in single-sex versus co-educational classroom settings. Eat Behav 2017;25:23–31.
49. Richardson SM, Paxton SJ. An evaluation of a body image intervention based on risk factors for body dissatisfaction: a controlled study with adolescent girls. Int J Eat Disord 2010;43:112–22.
50. McLean SA, Wertheim EH, Masters J, et al. A pilot evaluation of a social media literacy intervention to reduce risk factors for eating disorders. Int J Eat Disord 2017;50:847–51.
51. Turner H, Tatham M, Lant M, et al. Clinicians' concerns about delivering cognitive-behavioural therapy for eating disorders. Behav Res Ther 2014;57:38–42.
52. Cash TF. The body image workbook. An eight-step program for learning to like your looks. Oakland (CA): New Harbinger Publications, Inc; 2008.
53. McLean SA, Paxton SJ, Wertheim EH. A body image and disordered eating intervention for women in midlife: a randomized controlled trial. J Consult Clin Psychol 2011;79:751–8.

54. Paxton SJ, McLean SA, Gollings EK, et al. Comparison of face-to-face and Internet interventions for body image and eating problems in adult women: an RCT. Int J Eat Disord 2007;40:692–704.

55. Paxton SJ, McLean SA. Treatment for body-image disturbances. In: Grilo CM, Mitchell JE, editors. The treatment of eating disorders: a clinical handbook. New York: Guilford Press; 2010. p. 471–86.

56. Alleva JM, Sheeran P, Webb TL, et al. A meta-analytic review of stand-alone interventions to improve body image. PLoS One 2015;10:e0139177.

57. Walker DC, White EK, Srinivasan VJ. A meta-analysis of the relationships between body checking, body image avoidance, body image dissatisfaction, mood, and disordered eating. International Journal of Eating Disorders, Advance online publication 2018.

58. Reas DL, Grilo CM, Masheb RM, et al. Body checking and avoidance in overweight patients with binge eating disorder. Int J Eat Disord 2005;37:342–6.

59. Trentowska M, Svaldi J, Tuschen-Caffier B. Efficacy of body exposure as treatment component for patients with eating disorders. J Behav Ther Exp Psychiatry 2014;45:178–85.

60. Albertson ER, Neff KD, Dill-Shackleford KE. Self-compassion and body dissatisfaction in women: a randomized controlled trial of a brief meditation intervention. Mindfulness 2015;6:444–54.

61. Pacanowski CR, Diers L, Crosby RD, et al. Yoga in the treatment of eating disorders within a residential program: a randomized controlled trial. Eat Disord 2017; 25:37–51.

62. Ciao AC, Loth K, Neumark-Sztainer D. Preventing eating disorder pathology: common and unique features of successful eating disorders prevention programs. Curr Psychiatry Rep 2014;16:1–13.

63. Atkinson MJ, Wade T. Mindfulness-based prevention for eating disorders: a school-based cluster randomized controlled study. Int J Eat Disord 2015;48: 1024–37.

64. Rodgers RF, Donovan E, Cousineau T, et al. BodiMojo: efficacy of a mobile-based intervention in improving body image and self-compassion among adolescents. J Youth Adolesc 2018;47:1363–72.

65. Brown TA, Forney KJ, Pinner D, et al. A randomized controlled trial of The Body Project: more than muscles for men with body dissatisfaction. Int J Eat Disord 2017;50:873–83.

66. Swenne I. Influence of premorbid BMI on clinical characteristics at presentation of adolescent girls with eating disorders. BMC Psychiatry 2016;16:81.

Feeding and Eating Disorders in Children

Rachel Bryant-Waugh, BSc, MSc, DPhil[a,b]

KEYWORDS

- ARFID • Avoidant/restrictive food intake disorder
- Feeding and eating disorders of childhood

KEY POINTS

- All 6 of the formal feeding and eating disorders (pica, rumination disorder, avoidant-restrictive food intake disorder, anorexia nervosa, bulimia nervosa and binge eating disorder) may develop in childhood.
- Differentiation between transient feeding and eating difficulties likely to resolve over time and clinically significant disorders is essential to optimizing children's health, development, and well-being.
- Children with feeding and eating disorders require multiprofessional evaluation and management and family-centered models of care.
- Further research is needed to improve knowledge about the epidemiology, characterization, course, and outcome of these disorders in children.

INTRODUCTION

Feeding and eating difficulties are not uncommon during childhood and are often regarded as part of normal development. Many parents report that their children go through difficult phases that can broadly be differentiated into undereating, overeating, and fussy or faddy eating. In the majority of children, such episodes do not reach clinical significance and tend to resolve over time.[1] Management is typically conservative, incorporating reassurance, advice, and follow-up as indicated.[2] For some children, however, problematic eating patterns reach a clinical threshold and constitute a formal feeding or eating disorder, whereas in others, eating difficulties become established habits that may predispose to later eating or weight difficulties.[3,4]

Disclosure Statement: No disclosures to declare of any relationship with a commercial company that has a direct financial interest in subject matter or materials discussed in article or with a company making a competing product.
[a] Department of Child and Adolescent Mental Health, Great Ormond Street Hospital for Children NHS Foundation Trust, Great Ormond Street, London, WC1N 3JH, UK; [b] Population, Policy and Practice Programme, University College London Institute of Child Health, 30 Guilford Street, WC1N 1EH, London, UK
E-mail address: r.bryant-waugh@ucl.ac.uk

Psychiatr Clin N Am 42 (2019) 157–167
https://doi.org/10.1016/j.psc.2018.10.005
0193-953X/19/© 2018 Elsevier Inc. All rights reserved.

Abbreviations	
AN	Anorexia nervosa
ARFID	Avoidant/restrictive food intake disorder
BED	Binge eating disorder
BN	Bulimia nervosa
DSM-IV	*Diagnostic and Statistical Manual of Mental Disorders*, 4th edition
ICD	*International Classification of Diseases*
RD	Rumination disorder

The establishment of adequate food intake and eating behavior is fundamental to optimizing children's social, emotional, and cognitive development as well as their physical health and development, making this an important focus for attention. The identification of formal feeding and eating disorders may be missed in children, a situation that is widely acknowledged to require improvement.[5] Clinically significant feeding and eating disturbances are most common in children who have other medical, developmental, emotional, or behavioral difficulties, requiring all clinicians working with this age group to be alert to their possible presence. This article provides an update based on recently published literature and expert consensus on the current state of knowledge regarding feeding and eating disorders in children aged 2 to 12 years. It does not include discussion of infant feeding problems or disorders occurring in adolescence.

DIAGNOSIS

Until recently, there was a clear distinction between childhood feeding disorders and typically later onset eating disorders in psychiatric diagnostic classification. In the American Psychiatric Association's *Diagnostic and Statistical Manual of Mental Disorders*, 4th edition (DSM-IV), the section Feeding and Eating Disorders of Infancy or Early Childhood included pica, rumination disorder (RD), and feeding disorder of infancy or early childhood.[6] Given that it is well-known that pica and RD can also develop in older individuals, to include adults, the placement of these 2 disorders in a section for Disorders Usually First Diagnosed in Infancy, Childhood, or Adolescence was inconsistent with clinical reality. Furthermore, the DSM-IV diagnostic category feeding disorder of infancy or early childhood was overly broad and nonspecific, and only very rarely used in research studies. It also excluded children in whom the onset of eating difficulties was over the age of 6 years.

Clinicians working with children had long described the difficulties they experienced in assigning diagnoses to the clinically significant presentations of childhood eating disturbances that they were seeing and had developed a range of terms to describe their patients.[7–9] Unfortunately, this strategy resulted in a plethora of descriptive labels with a lack of standardization regarding their use. Such a situation undoubtedly hampers research, to include treatment research; without universally agreed on and accepted diagnostic criteria, investigators cannot be sure that they are including similar patients. The field of childhood-onset feeding and eating disorders has arguably struggled as a consequence in making significant progress in matching specific clinical presentations to best evidence-based treatments.

With the publication of DSM-5 in 2013,[10] and subsequently in the World Health Organization's *International Classification of Diseases* (ICD), updated and published in 2018 in the form of ICD-11,[11] the feeding and eating disorder diagnoses have been reworked and brought together under 1 heading. Both of these revised and updated classification systems have moved away from disorders being classified by typical age of onset, in line with evidence suggesting that core psychopathology across a range of disorders is often consistent, but may be differently expressed by individuals at different stages of development. In both the DSM-5 and the ICD-11, the criteria for feeding disorder of infancy or early childhood have been reworded and extended on the basis of published evidence and existing data, and renamed avoidant/restrictive food intake disorder (ARFID). This category now encompasses some of the clinical presentations commonly seen in childhood, but previously failing to fit available criteria for feeding and eating disorders. This step forward is significant, in particular for diagnostic practice in children.

Owing to the coming together under 1 heading and the developmental emphasis incorporated in wording, the 6 formal feeding and eating disorder categories in DSM-5 and ICD-11 are all potentially applicable to presentations of eating disturbance in childhood. There are documented cases of all 6 disorders, namely, pica, RD, ARFID, anorexia nervosa (AN), bulimia nervosa (BN), and binge eating disorder (BED) in individuals younger than 13 years of age.[12–17] Pica, RD, ARFID, and AN are the disorders most commonly encountered by clinicians working with children presenting with eating disturbances. BN and BED are less commonly seen because these disorders typically have an adolescent or adult onset. Each disorder is discussed briefly in turn in relation to clinical features specific to children. Reliable incidence and prevalence data for this age range are scarce and are mentioned where relevant.

Pica

Pica, defined as the regular eating of nonfood, nonnutritive substances, is perhaps most commonly encountered by clinicians working with children in those with intellectual disability. It is also seen in children with specific sensory needs, for example, those who seek oral stimulation, which may include children on the autism spectrum. However, pica can also occur in normally developing children and the possibility of this behavior being present is often overlooked in routine clinical assessment. The etiology of pica in children is most likely to be multifactorial and to vary between individuals, but may include exploratory behavior, self-stimulation or seeking sensory feedback, self-soothing, or nutritional deficiencies.

Owing to the ingestion of substances or items that are potentially toxic, harmful, and typically indigestible, pica can have serious medical consequences. These consequences may include poisoning, abdominal perforation, blockages, or the formation of bezoars; in some cases, the behavior can have fatal consequences.[18] Despite this risk, there are few studies investigating its incidence and prevalence in children. A recent population-based study in Germany, which included 804 children aged 7 to 14 years and their parents, found that pica behavior was reported to have occurred at least once in 12.3% of children, with recurring pica behavior reported in 5%.[19] In terms of treatment, current advice continues to focus predominantly on behavioral interventions and appropriate management of the environment.[20,21] There is limited evidence for the use of medication for the treatment of pica in children.[22]

Rumination Disorder

RD is defined as the repeated regurgitation of food, followed by rechewing and reswallowing or spitting out. This should be differentiated from gastroesophageal reflux or vomiting with a primary medical cause. Manometry, in particular high-resolution esophageal manometry, may assist in the diagnosis of RD,[23] but a careful history and clinical observation may suffice in more straightforward presentations. The regurgitation in RD occurs without undue effort with the process of bringing food back up into the mouth, rechewing and swallowing or spitting often being experienced as pleasurable. As with pica, it is most commonly seen by the clinician working with children in those with learning disabilities and other developmental disorders. It can also occur in children who have suffered abuse or neglect, as well as in normally developing children with largely unremarkable histories aside from temperamental anxiety. Often, RD behaviors can be quite subtle and may be missed; however, in other cases the behavior is very obvious and can cause marked impairment to everyday functioning. Children with RD may present as underweight and malnourished, although this is not always the case. In extreme cases, the constant bringing up of food may result in emaciation and the need for enteral feeding, to include percutaneous endoscopic gastrojejunostomy feeding. Signs of RD include a persistent smell of stomach acid and dental decay through erosion of tooth enamel. Again, the etiology is most likely to vary and be multifactorial. RD typically presents as an habitual behavior, often increasing in intensity when the child experiences stress or anxiety.

The incidence and prevalence of RD in children remains poorly researched. The German population-based study mentioned identified slightly lower rates of reported RD than of pica: in the study population of 804 children aged 7 to 14 years and their parents, RD behavior was reported to have occurred at least once in 11.5% of children, with recurring RD behavior reported in 1.5%.[19] Current treatment recommendations include behavioral approaches, to include habit reversal training, as well as cognitive–behavioral approaches for older children able to access this form of therapy. Again, there is limited evidence for pharmacologic treatment and this modality is not generally recommended as a first-line intervention.

Avoidant/Restrictive Food Intake Disorder

ARFID is characterized by avoidant or restrictive eating behavior that may be linked to a number of different underlying features. The best characterized presentations are reflected in the examples given in the DSM-5 diagnostic criteria, namely those with low interest in food and eating, those whose avoidance is primarily related to sensory issues, and those in whom restriction or avoidance is predominantly fear related.[10]

Children with ARFID may present with 1 or more of these underlying features, because they are not mutually exclusive and these examples do not constitute separate subgroups, at least as far as we know from existing evidence. The eating disturbance is associated with insufficient intake in terms of the individual's overall energy needs and/or their nutritional requirements in terms of food groups and micronutrients. Individuals with ARFID may be underweight, normal weight, or overweight. In children with ARFID, growth velocity may be adversely affected. Because ARFID is a relatively newly defined diagnostic category, there is much still to learn. Research interest is growing with appropriate greater involvement of both feeding disorder and eating disorder professionals. At this stage, it seems important to continue to conceptualize ARFID as an "umbrella" diagnosis; further refinement of our understanding and knowledge about the disorder and potential subtypes should emerge over the coming years.

Robust population-based incidence and prevalence rates for a confirmed diagnosis of ARFID in children remain to be established. In a study seeking to identify the distribution of avoidant and restrictive eating behaviors characteristic of ARFID, 1444 schoolchildren in Switzerland aged 8 to 13 years were screened.[24] The children were invited to complete a newly developed self-report measure, the Eating Disturbances in Youth-Questionnaire, which includes items based on the DSM-5 diagnostic criteria. Findings revealed that 46 of the 1442 children (3.2%) reported ARFID features. Of these children, 28 (60.9%) identified sensory properties of food as contributing to their avoidance, 18 (39.1%) identified low interest in food or eating, and 7 (15.2%)

identified a fear-based reason for food avoidance, such as a fear of vomiting or choking.[24]

Other studies have investigated ARFID rates within specific clinical populations, with the most frequently studied to date being child and adolescent eating disorder programs. For example, a Canadian study that included patients under the age of 18 years attending a pediatric tertiary care eating disorders program found that of 369 patients assessed, 31 (8.4%) were given a diagnosis of ARFID after assessment compared with 274 (74.3%) given a diagnosis of AN. Of those with ARFID, 11 (35.5%) were under the age of 12 years, with presentations in the overwhelming majority associated with low weight.[14] A chart review study of 7- to 17-year-old children admitted to a day program in the United States identified a greater proportion of patients with ARFID, although these diagnoses were retrospectively conferred: of a total of 173 patients, 39 (22.5%) had a diagnosis of ARFID compared with 53.8% with AN. Of note is the finding that the mean age of the ARFID patients was 11.1 years with a standard deviation of 1.7, which was significantly younger than the mean age of AN patients at 14.0 years (standard deviation = 1.5).[25] The finding that in eating disorder programs, ARFID patients tend to be on average younger and include more males that other diagnostic groups seems to be relatively consistent. Higher rates of cooccurring conditions, including anxiety disorders, developmental disorders, and learning disorders, have also been identified within ARFID patients compared with those with other eating disorders.

The key characteristic of avoidance or restriction has been proposed as existing on a continuum from normal to abnormal in terms of children's eating behaviors. A study based on mealtime observations of 18 children with a diagnosis of ARFID and 21 children with no disordered eating identified common behaviors across both groups. Significant group differences were noted in the frequency of food intake behaviors, engagement with feeding, and restlessness during mealtimes.[26] The suggestion put forward by the investigating team on the basis of these findings is that clinicians should focus on child engagement with food and restlessness during mealtimes in the identification of ARFID in this age group, rather than focus exclusively on the type of behavior exhibited.

There are currently a small number of treatment studies with patients with ARFID under way, predominantly focusing on adolescents and young adults. However, one randomized controlled cross-over trial is focusing exclusively on 5- to 12-year-old children with ARFID, testing the feasibility and acceptability of a novel intervention, Family Based Treatment of ARFID in this age group.[27,28] Other than this, there is a large body of literature on the treatment of pediatric feeding disorders, much of which may be relevant to ARFID. Behavioral approaches are the most commonly cited as helpful, and represent the main empirically supported therapy for feeding disorders in children.[29]

Pharmacologic treatments have also been described as potentially helpful in children with ARFID or related restrictive eating difficulties, but always as an adjunctive treatment only. For example, olanzapine in low-dose administration has been reported to facilitate eating, weight gain, and the reduction of anxious, depressive, and cognitive symptoms in children with ARFID[30] and cyproheptadine has been identified as safe and effective for use in young children with eating difficulties related to low appetite, in combination with specialized multidisciplinary intervention.[31] One further recent study included 15 young children with ARFID (aged 20–58 months) using a double-blind, placebo-controlled trial comparing behavioral intervention with behavioral intervention plus D-cycloserine, which has been shown to assist in exposure interventions in anxiety disorders.[32] The authors conclude that the positive results noted in terms of improvements to eating behavior warrant a larger scale study of D-cycloserine for the treatment of pediatric feeding problems, to include ARFID.

Anorexia Nervosa

The existence of AN in children, or AN with a prepubertal onset, has long been recognized, with examples of early onset male and female cases reported from around the world.[33,34] Children with AN must meet the same diagnostic criteria as adolescents and adults for the diagnosis to be conferred, although some differences in presentation and course have been identified. In 1 study comparing 30 children with early onset AN and 30 patients with adolescent onset AN, the younger patients were found to share the same core psychopathology and to have similar hospitalization rates and levels of body image distortion as the older patients. However, they were also found to have required more tube feeding and to display more restrictive eating behavior, but experience fewer problems with self-esteem and perfectionism.[35] However, these findings were not replicated in another study comparing cognitive, behavioral, and physical and medical features of children ($\leq$12 years) and adolescents (13–18 years) with eating disorders, although this study did not focus specifically on AN.[36]

The incidence and prevalence rates of early or childhood onset AN are harder to determine and are often presented along with adolescent onset data.[37] There is some indication that the age at onset of AN may be decreasing,[38,39] suggesting that childhood presentations of AN may increase as a consequence. In terms of those accessing treatment, children under the age of 13 years currently represent a much smaller group than adolescent patients. For example, in a German registry study of young people receiving in-patient care for AN, 10.5% of 258 hospitalized patients aged 8 to 18 included in the study were under the age of 12 years.[40]

First-line recommended treatment for AN in children includes medical monitoring and management, family-based psychological intervention, and supplementary dietary advice all with an emphasis on ensuring that growth and development needs are met.[41] Medication is not typically recommended as a primary treatment, but may serve a useful adjunctive role in the management of cooccurring anxiety or mood disorders.

The evidence about longer term outcomes in this age group is inconsistent. It is most likely that children developing AN may show a similar spectrum of outcomes as older onset patients, ranging from full remission to poor outcomes. A recent study set out to investigate outcomes in patients with onset of AN before the age of 14. Sixty-eight participants were followed for an average of 7.5 years after admission, with a minimum follow-up period of 4.5 years. Of these, 52 subjects with a mean age of 12.5 years at onset (standard deviation = 1.0) were assessed further, revealing that approximately 41% had a good outcome, 35% an intermediate outcome, and 24% had a poor outcome. At follow-up, 28% met the current criteria for another psychiatric disorder and 64% had a past psychiatric disorder. The authors identified only higher weight at admission as a positive outcome predictor and conclude that childhood onset AN is a serious disorder with relatively high rates of unfavorable outcomes and cooccurring psychiatric disorders.[42]

Bulimia Nervosa and Binge Eating Disorder

Childhood presentations of formally diagnosed BN and BED are less commonly seen in clinical settings than the other eating disorders. For example, in a UK surveillance study of children under the age of 13 years presenting to secondary care for treatment of an eating disorder, 37% met criteria for AN whereas only 1.4% met criteria for BN.[43] Evidence suggests that BN typically has an adolescent or young adult onset, with BED a slightly higher peak age of onset. However, there has been some suggestion that age at onset of BN seems to be decreasing,[39] but this finding is not consistent, with other studies showing a decrease in age at onset of AN but not BN.[38] A recent US study identified median age at onset for DSM-IV BN as 12.4 years (interquartile range, 11.1–13.5 years),[44] which is certainly relatively young compared with earlier studies.

In children, there has been significant interest in loss-of-control eating, which has been identified as a risk factor for excess weight gain and BED. Family-based approaches addressing the interpersonal and emotional underpinnings of this type of eating in children have been proposed as showing promise in terms of prevention.[4] However, as with many areas in relation to childhood feeding and eating disturbances, further research is needed to be able to demonstrate this finding. In terms of first-line treatment guidance for children with BN, family-based psychological interventions with medical monitoring and management are generally recommended.[41]

DISCUSSION

Feeding and eating difficulties in children may have multiple contributing factors, to include factors specific to the child as well as factors related to parental management. We also know that having a child with a feeding or eating difficulty can be experienced as very stressful for primary caregivers and can adversely affect family relationships.[45,46] Disrupted interactions and mealtime stress can exacerbate and perpetuate difficulties. Irrespective of the nature of the difficulty and its onset, that is, whether the eating disturbance has been present from very early in feeding development or has a later onset relating to a specific aversive trigger, the existing literature highlights the need for comprehensive assessment and family-centered models of care to be considered.[14,47,48]

Children with feeding and eating disturbances therefore typically require multiprofessional input to ensure appropriate assessment and management. Disciplines commonly contributing to the comprehensive care of children with feeding and eating disorders include staff from pediatric medicine, nutrition and dietetics, speech and language pathology, psychology, psychiatry, occupational therapy, and nursing. The child's medical and developmental history require evaluation in terms of potential impact on appetite and eating behavior, as do the child's emotional and behavioral functioning, interactions around food, mealtime management, and family attitudes and practices and influences in relation to feeding. Oromotor control, the ability to swallow, and sensory issues are all familiar areas of consideration by pediatric medical staff working with children with feeding problems, given the potential for difficulties in these functions to interfere with normal feeding.[2] Mental health clinicians and those working in psychiatric or psychology clinics need to be alert to the possibility that such issues may be playing a role in a child's eating difficulty and liaise or refer on as needed. Consensus opinion, position statements, and reviews of studies of interventions for pediatric feeding disorders all indicate that multidisciplinary treatment holds greatest benefit.[29,49,50]

SUMMARY AND FUTURE DIRECTIONS

- All the formal feeding and eating disorder diagnoses can be found in children. Despite this, there continues to be relatively poor knowledge about the specific prevalence and incidence of these disorders in children under the age of 13 years.
- Historical differences in diagnostic practice and clinical terminology as well as the split between the fields of feeding disorders and eating disorders, both

clinically and academically, have hampered research. Much better characterization of these disorders, to include identification of common correlates, potential subgroups, and response to standardized, evidence-based treatment interventions is required.

- Feeding and eating disorders in children are most likely to have a multifactorial etiology, with variation in contributing factors between individuals. Common etiologic pathways require further elucidation and at the level of individual patients, clinicians need a range of evidence-based, robust assessment tools.
- Feeding and eating disorders in children require multiprofessional evaluation and management. This need has implications for screening, diagnosis, referral pathways, service design, and delivery of clinical care. Optimal arrangements for clinical practice require development and evaluation.
- Current best evidence for feeding disorders in children is for behavioral approaches and for eating disorders is a family-based intervention, both in conjunction with medical and dietetic monitoring and management. There is limited evidence for pharmacologic management, which is never recommended as a first-line treatment, but may be useful as an adjunctive intervention. Parental involvement in treatment is always required.

REFERENCES

1. Cardona Cano S, Tiemeier H, Van Hoeken D, et al. Trajectories of picky eating during childhood: a general population study. Int J Eat Disord 2015;48:570–9.
2. Borowitz KC, Borowitz SM. Feeding problems in infants and children: assessment and etiology. Pediatr Clin North Am 2018;65:59–72.
3. Jacobi C, Hayward C, de Zwaan M, et al. Coming to terms with risk factors for eating disorders: application of risk terminology and suggestions for a general taxonomy. Psychol Bull 2004;130:19–65.
4. Shomaker LB, Tanofsky-Kraff M, Matherne CE, et al. A randomized, comparative pilot trial of family-based interpersonal psychotherapy for reducing psychosocial symptoms, disordered-eating, and excess weight gain in at-risk preadolescents with loss-of-control-eating. Int J Eat Disord 2017;50:1084–94.
5. Sacco B, Kelley U. Diagnosis and evaluation of eating disorders in the pediatric patient. Pediatr Ann 2018;47:e244–9.
6. American Psychiatric Association. Diagnostic and statistical manual of mental disorders, 4th edition, text revision (DSM-IV-TR). Washington (DC): American Psychiatric Publishing; 2000.
7. Nicholls D, Chater R, Lask B. Children into DSM don't go: a comparison of classification systems for eating disorders in childhood and early adolescence. Int J Eat Disord 2000;28:317–24.
8. Bryant-Waugh R, Lask B. Overview of eating disorders in childhood and adolescence. In: Lask B, Bryant-Waugh R, editors. Eating disorders in childhood and adolescence. 4th edition. London: Routledge; 2013. p. 33–49.
9. Chatoor I. Diagnosis and treatment of feeding disorders in infants, toddlers and young children. Washington (DC): Zero to Three; 2009.
10. American Psychiatric Association. Diagnostic and statistical manual of mental disorders. 5th edition. Arlington (VA: American Psychiatric Publishing; 2013.
11. World Health Organisation. International classification of diseases, 11th Revision (ICD-11). Available at: http://www.who.int/classifications/icd/en/. Accessed August 15, 2018.

12. Miao D, Young SL, Golden CD. A meta-analysis of pica and micronutrient status. Am J Hum Biol 2015;27:84–93.
13. Raha B, Sarma S, Thilakan P, et al. Rumination disorder: an unexplained case of recurrent vomiting. Indian J Psychol Med 2017;39:361–3.
14. Cooney M, Lieberman M, Guimond T, et al. Clinical and psychological features of children and adolescents diagnosed with avoidant/restrictive food intake disorder in a pediatric tertiary care eating disorder program: a descriptive study. J Eat Disord 2018;6:7.
15. Holland J, Hall N, Yeates DGR, et al. Trends in hospital admission rates for anorexia nervosa in Oxford (1968–2011) and England (1990–2011): database studies. J R Soc Med 2016;109:59–66.
16. Day J, Schmidt U, Collier D, et al. Risk factors, correlates, and markers in early-onset bulimia nervosa and EDNOS. Int J Eat Disord 2010;44:287–94.
17. Shapiro JR, Woolson SL, Hamer RM, et al. Evaluating binge eating disorder in children: development of the children's binge eating disorder scale (C-BEDS). Int J Eat Disord 2007;40:82–9.
18. Matejů E, Duchanová S, Kovac P, et al. Fatal case of Rapunzel syndrome in neglected child. Forensic Sci Int 2009;190:e5–7.
19. Hartmann AS, Poulain T, Vogel M, et al. Prevalence of pica and rumination behaviors in German children aged 7-14 and their associations with feeding, eating, and general psychopathology: a population-based study. Eur Child Adolesc Psychiatry 2018. https://doi.org/10.1007/s00787-018-1153-9.
20. Saini V, Greer BD, Fisher WW, et al. Individual and combined effects of noncontingent reinforcement and response blocking on automatically reinforced problem behavior. J Appl Behav Anal 2016;49:693–8.
21. Hauptman M, Woolf AD. Childhood ingestions of environmental toxins: what are the risks? Pediatr Ann 2017;46:e466–71.
22. McNaughten B, Bourke T, Thompson A. Fifteen-minute consultation: the child with pica. Arch Dis Child Educ Pract Ed 2017;102:226–9.
23. Righini Grunder F, Aspirot A, Faure C. High-resolution esophageal manometry patterns in children and adolescents with rumination syndrome. J Pediatr Gastroenterol Nutr 2017;65:627–32.
24. Kurz S, van Dyck Z, Dremmel D, et al. Early-onset restrictive eating disturbances in primary school boys and girls. Eur Child Adolesc Psychiatry 2015;24:779–85.
25. Nicely TA, Lane-Loney S, Masciulli E, et al. Prevalence and characteristics of avoidant/restrictive food intake disorder in a cohort of young patients in day treatment for eating disorders. J Eat Disord 2014;2:21.
26. Aldridge VK, Dovey TM, El Hawi N, et al. Observation and comparison of mealtime behaviors in a sample of children with avoidant/restrictive food intake disorders and a control sample of children with typical development. Infant Ment Health J 2018;39:410–22.
27. Lock J. Treating ARFID using family-based treatment: a randomized controlled crossover trial. Available at: https://www.nationaleatingdisorders.org/ways-to-give/feeding-hope-fund-clinical-research/recipients/. Accessed August 15, 2018.
28. Rienecke RD. Family based treatment of eating disorders in adolescents: current insights. Adolesc Health Med Ther 2017;8:69–79.
29. Morris N, Knight RM, Bruni T, et al. Feeding disorders. Child Adolesc Psychiatr Clin N Am 2017;26:571–86.
30. Brewerton TD, D'Agostino M. Adjunctive use of olanzapine in the treatment of avoidant/restrictive food intake disorder in children and adolescents in an eating disorders program. J Child Adolesc Psychopharmacol 2017;27:920–2.

31. Sant'Anna AM, Hammes PS, Porporino M, et al. Use of cyproheptadine in young children with feeding difficulties and poor growth in a pediatric feeding program. J Pediatr Gastroenterol Nutr 2014;59:674–8.
32. Sharp WG, Allen AG, Stubbs KH, et al. Successful pharmacotherapy for the treatment of severe feeding aversion with mechanistic insights from cross-species neuronal remodelling. Transl Psychiatry 2017;7:1157.
33. Vijayvergia D, Sharma DK, Agarwal S, et al. Anorexia Nervosa-restricted type with obsessive traits in a pre-pubertal female: a case report. Indian J Psychiatry 2012; 54:392–3.
34. Berksoy EA, Özyurt G, Anıl M, et al. Can pediatricians recognize eating disorders? A case study of early-onset anorexia nervosa in a male child. Nutr Hosp 2018;27:499–502.
35. van Noort BM, Lohmar SK, Pfeiffer E, et al. Clinical characteristics of early onset anorexia nervosa. Eur Eat Disord Rev 2018;26(5):519–25.
36. Walker T, Watson HJ, Leach DJ, et al. Comparative study of children and adolescents referred for eating disorder treatment at a specialist tertiary setting. Int J Eat Disord 2014;47:47–53.
37. Jaite C, Hoffmann F, Glaeske G, et al. Prevalence, comorbidities and outpatient treatment of anorexia and bulimia nervosa in German children and adolescents. Eat Weight Disord 2013;18:157–65.
38. Steinhausen HC, Jensen CM. Time trends in lifetime incidence rates of first-time diagnosed anorexia nervosa and bulimia nervosa across 16 years in a Danish nationwide psychiatric registry study. Int J Eat Disord 2015;48:845–50.
39. Favaro A, Caregaro L, Tenconi E, et al. Time trends in age at onset of anorexia nervosa and bulimia nervosa. J Clin Psychiatry 2009;70:1715–21.
40. Bühren K, Herpertz-Dahlmann B, Dempfle A, et al. First sociodemographic, pretreatment and clinical data from a German web-based registry for child and adolescent anorexia nervosa. Z Kinder Jugendpsychiatr Psychother 2017;45: 393–400.
41. National Institute for Health and Care Excellence. Eating disorders: recognition and treatment. 2017. Available at: https://www.nice.org.uk/guidance/ng69. Accessed August 15, 2018.
42. Herpertz-Dahlmann B, Dempfle A, Egberts KM, et al. Outcome of childhood anorexia nervosa-The results of a five- to ten-year follow-up study. Int J Eat Disord 2018;51:295–304.
43. Nicholls DE, Lynn R, Viner RM. Childhood eating disorders: British National Surveillance Study. Br J Psychiatry 2011;198:295–301.
44. Hail L, Le Grange D. Bulimia nervosa in adolescents: prevalence and treatment challenges. Adolesc Health Med Ther 2018;9:11–6.
45. Jones CJ, Bryant-Waugh R. The relationship between child feeding problems and maternal mental health: a selective review. Adv Eat Disord 2013;1:119–33.
46. Aviram I, Atzaba-Poria N, Pike A, et al. Mealtime dynamics in child feeding disorder: the role of child temperament, parental sense of competence and paternal involvement. J Pediatr Psychol 2015;40:45–54.
47. DerMarderosian D, Chapman HA, Tortolani C, et al. Medical considerations in children and adolescents with eating disorders. Child Adolesc Psychiatry Clin N Am 2018;27:1–14.
48. Follent AM, Rumbach AF, Ward EC, et al. Dysphagia and feeding difficulties postpediatric ingestion injury: perspectives of the primary caregiver. Int J Pediatr Otorhinolaryngol 2017;103:20–8.

49. Sharp WG, Volkert VM, Scahill L, et al. A systematic review and meta-analysis of intensive multidisciplinary intervention for pediatric feeding disorders: how standard is the standard of care? J Pediatr 2017;181:116–24.
50. The British Academy of Childhood Disability. Pathway for children with feeding problems. Available at: https://www.bacdis.org.uk/policy/documents/feedingpathway.pdf. Accessed August 15, 2018.

Moving?

Make sure your subscription moves with you!

To notify us of your new address, find your **Clinics Account Number** (located on your mailing label above your name), and contact customer service at:

Email: **journalscustomerservice-usa@elsevier.com**

800-654-2452 (subscribers in the U.S. & Canada)
314-447-8871 (subscribers outside of the U.S. & Canada)

Fax number: **314-447-8029**

Elsevier Health Sciences Division
Subscription Customer Service
3251 Riverport Lane
Maryland Heights, MO 63043

*To ensure uninterrupted delivery of your subscription, please notify us at least 4 weeks in advance of move.

Moving?

Make sure your subscription moves with you!

To notify us of your new address, find your Clinics Account Number (located on your mailing label above your name), and contact customer service at:

Email: JournalsCustomerService-usa@elsevier.com

800-654-2452 (subscribers in the U.S. & Canada)
314-447-8871 (subscribers outside of the U.S. & Canada)

Fax number: 314-447-8029

Elsevier Health Sciences Division
Subscription Customer Service
3251 Riverport Lane
Maryland Heights, MO 63043

Printed and bound by CPI Group (UK) Ltd, Croydon, CR0 4YY

03/10/2024

01040479-0017